Using Acceptance and Commitment Therapy with Adults with Intellectual Disabilities

of related interest

Love, Learning Disabilities and Pockets of Brilliance
How Practitioners Can Make a Difference to the
Lives of Children, Families and Adults
Sara Ryan
ISBN 978 1 78775 191 0
eISBN 978 1 78775 192 7

**Preventing the Emotional Abuse and Neglect of
People with Intellectual Disability**
Stopping Insult and Injury
Sally Robinson
ISBN 978 1 84905 230 6
eISBN 978 0 85700 472 7

ACT Art Therapy
Creative Approaches to Acceptance and Commitment Therapy
Dr Amy Backos
ISBN 978 1 78775 803 2
eISBN 978 1 78775 804 9

Using Acceptance and Commitment Therapy with Adults with Intellectual Disabilities

Dr Sarah Tomlinson,
Dr Jonathan Williams
and Dr Natalie Boulton

Jessica Kingsley Publishers
London and Philadelphia

First published in Great Britain in 2025 by Jessica Kingsley Publishers
An imprint of John Murray Press

2

Copyright © Sarah Tomlinson, Jonathan Williams and Natalie Boulton 2025

The right of Sarah Tomlinson, Jonathan Williams and Natalie Boulton
to be identified as the Author of the Work has been asserted by them in
accordance with the Copyright, Designs and Patents Act 1988.

Figure 2.1 The Hexaflex reproduced by kind permission of Steven Hayes
Figure 2.5 The Choice Point reproduced by kind permission of Russ Harris

A CIP catalogue record for this title is available from the
British Library and the Library of Congress

ISBN 978 1 80501 299 3
eISBN 978 1 80501 300 6

Printed and bound in the United States by Integrated Books International

Jessica Kingsley Publishers' policy is to use papers that are natural,
renewable and recyclable products and made from wood grown in
sustainable forests. The logging and manufacturing processes are expected
to conform to the environmental regulations of the country of origin.

Jessica Kingsley Publishers
Carmelite House
50 Victoria Embankment
London EC4Y 0DZ

www.jkp.com

John Murray Press
Part of Hodder & Stoughton Limited
An Hachette UK Company

The authorized representative in the EEA is Hachette Ireland,
8 Castlecourt Centre, Dublin 15, D15 XTP3, Ireland (email: info@hbgi.ie)

Contents

Conclusion: Where do we go from here? 212

Introduction

Our 'raison d'être' as clinical psychologists is to contribute towards improving the lives of people with intellectual disabilities in a meaningful way. Acceptance and Commitment Therapy (ACT) has had a profound impact upon our practice. In collaboration with each person's support networks, it has helped to create more fulfilling lives for many people. We hope that in writing this book we will help other practitioners to move towards the same outcome. We have found that ACT has something unique and valuable to offer people with intellectual disabilities and their wider support network. ACT provides a framework to effect change in several ways. We want to share how that can be done.

A wealth of incredibly helpful material is available to enable a practitioner to use ACT with the general population. There are evidence-based protocols that target specific challenges and disorders such as anxiety, depression, anger and eating difficulties. There is also strong evidence to support the use of ACT for chronic pain, and it is recommended by the UK National Institute for Health and Care Excellence (NICE, 2021). However, little has been written about ACT for people with intellectual disabilities. There are just a handful of studies, primarily case studies, and no randomized-controlled trials, making it difficult to generalize the findings more widely. Even less is available with respect to books. Two exceptions are: *Living Your Best Life* (Williams & Jones, 2022), a guided self-help resource that, to our knowledge, is the only published ACT book written for people with intellectual disabilities, and *The Art of Caring for People with Intellectual Disabilities* by the same author team (Jones & Williams, 2023), which uses ACT concepts and principles and is for direct care providers of people with intellectual disabilities. We wrote this book to address this gap and demonstrate how intellectual disability practitioners can effectively use ACT with individuals with intellectual disabilities, and how they can support both paid and family supporters in their roles. We have preferred, in this book, to avoid the use of client or patient, and in keeping with the ACT philosophy of 'we are all in the same boat', we have simply referred to people, or people with intellectual disabilities.

The ACT model can be used for many issues affecting people with intellectual disabilities. For example, the Acceptance element of ACT can be useful in relation to unchangeable situations, and sadly, many people with intellectual disabilities have experienced numerous painful life experiences that cannot be changed. These may include the lifelong impact of having cognitive difficulties that often make it difficult to understand or manage everyday life independently; or living alongside other people not of their choosing, sometimes in a location far away from home that may never have been the preference. ACT can also be useful as a framework for coping with difficult thoughts and feelings in current situations, and many people with intellectual disabilities can have difficulty in regulating or understanding feelings. Supporters of people with intellectual disabilities may equally find challenges in coping with their own distress or that of the person with intellectual disability. (Of course, this is not an exhaustive list. Take the time to discover the things that have been difficult for the individual you are working alongside through collaborative formulation, covered in Chapter 2.)

To truly appreciate the experiences of people you are working with, we begin by considering the context and histories of the lives of people with intellectual disabilities. We hope this book will support the creative implementation of a range of ACT-inspired principles for practitioners working alongside people with intellectual disabilities and their supporters. We offer a process-based approach, which includes consideration of observable behaviours in session that may indicate whether or not a person is struggling with particular psychological skills (see Hoffman and Hayes, 2019, for further information about process-based approaches). These descriptions owe a huge debt to Wilson and DuFrene from the book *Mindfulness for Two* (2009), in which behavioural correlates with different processes are outlined, offering the ability to make an estimate of the person's skills and difficulties in the different areas of psychological skills within an ACT framework. In this book we adapt and summarize these ideas to inform the assessment and formulation phases of an ACT-based intervention and to inform the real-time monitoring of therapeutic progress. We also offer our thanks to Russ Harris, who developed the 'Choice Point' (Chapter 3) and generously gave us permission to adapt it for this book.

We hope that, as well as being informative, this book is also easy to read, with plenty of useful practical ideas and resources. We do not believe it is in the interest of people with intellectual disabilities to restrict access to useful resources, and we have therefore included various adapted materials for practitioners to use. Some of which can be downloaded from https://

digitalhub.jkp.com/redeem using the code UAHJYLC; alternatively, scan the QR code. To help bring to life how ACT can be applied, we have peppered the book with various (anonymized) case examples. This book does not outline a 'cookbook' stepwise approach. Instead, it offers building blocks: core principles and ways to adapt mainstream ACT approaches, along with some examples of ways this might be realized. We offer some 'starter' ideas, and some example resources, but we also hope to equip practitioners to make use of and adapt some of the excellent mainstream and readily available ACT textbooks.

Who is this book for?

This book is primarily designed as a resource for any practitioners working with people with intellectual disabilities (also referred to as learning disabilities in some countries, such as the United Kingdom). For an individual to meet the criteria for a diagnosis of intellectual disability, the following three factors must be present (British Psychological Society, 2015):

- cognitive difficulties as demonstrated by an assessed IQ score of under 70
- corresponding difficulties with adaptive day-to-day skills
- evidence that the difficulties were evident before the age of 18.

We keep this definition in mind when considering our adaptations.

Emerson and Baines (2010) estimate that up to 20 or 30 percent of people with intellectual disabilities also have autism. For such individuals, we will discuss therapeutic approaches that take account of typical autism traits such as sensory sensitivity, literality or need for predictability.

The principles and strategies described in this book may also be relevant to other populations, including those with learning *difficulties* that do not meet the criteria for a diagnosis of a global intellectual disability. They may be useful too for other types of cognitive impairment, such as neurological problems and dementia, albeit with further adaptation and tailored flexibly to meet individual needs.

Whilst our focus is on adults, there is no reason why the material in this book cannot be used when working with children. Some of the content may need to be further adapted to match the developmental age of the child, and to be more 'child friendly'. Although the direct material may require further adaptation for children, the sections about working with the wider system are generally equally relevant.

We acknowledge that our book draws primarily from a Western perspective, albeit that some themes are likely to be relevant in other cultural contexts. We also acknowledge that some of our discussions are focused on the UK, in particular Chapter 1, which outlines the contextual basis for our work. However, we believe that much of the content, particularly beyond Chapter 1, is applicable internationally.

Finally, we offer our thanks to people with intellectual disabilities for their patience. For too long, they have been forced to tolerate the intolerable. We hope in some small way we, and you, can play a part in changing that.

THE WIDER CONTEXT

Working effectively and ethically with people with intellectual disabilities to improve lives and wellbeing requires more than just consideration of how psychological and therapeutic interventions need to be adapted. A more holistic consideration incorporating historical and recent cultural context is required. It goes without saying that everyone's experience will vary according to their particular life circumstances, including considerations of geography, culture and religion; but there are broader contextual factors that require understanding. In this chapter we cover the impact of sociohistorical factors and models of care relating to people with an intellectual disability up to the present day, and also briefly consider intersectionality.

The context

The resilience of people with intellectual disabilities is striking when one considers the frequent, repeated challenges and traumatic episodes so many individuals have experienced (Jones & Williams, 2023). Individuals are coping daily with intellectual and/or sensory/information-processing differences and on top of this face societal stigma, awareness of difference, co-morbid physical health difficulties, and increased likelihood of deprivation, bullying and abuse (Jones & Williams, 2023). It is unsurprising, then, that people with intellectual disabilities experience a higher rate of mental health problems than the general population. Although prevalence studies give widely varying results due to methodological differences, Cooper et al. (2018) found the point prevalence of clinical diagnosis of mental health problems to be 40.9 percent, much higher than those observed in the general population. However, Singleton et al. (2001) estimated the prevalence as between 16 and 25 percent (Cooper et al. included problem behaviours within their sample, which may have erroneously inflated the percentage). Other prevalence studies have suggested people with intellectual disabilities are three to four times more likely to have mental health problems than people in the general population (Cooper et al., 2007; Sheehan et al., 2015).

In the West, the role and place of people with intellectual disabilities was significantly negatively impacted upon by the Industrial Revolution. Prior to that, a greater proportion lived in smaller agricultural communities with greater emphasis on manual work. Many people with intellectual disabilities would have found meaningful occupation, employment and a sense of belonging via farming or other similar tasks, alongside many other people in their communities (Delap, 2023). The Industrial Revolution necessitated a much more skilled workforce and placed emphasis on measurable output of production, leading to a decrease in valued roles for many people with ID.

Of course, people with a range of intellectual disabilities are very able to learn various skills. However, the focus on productivity meant that many individuals were overlooked for such positions. Instead, an emphasis on institutional support grew, such as so-called 'poor houses' for people who were not able to work in industrialized settings for various reasons. These included many people with intellectual disabilities. And so began a cultural context of people being 'cared for' (although sometimes inadequately, if not abusively) rather than being fully integrated into wider society. This led to an erosion of the concept of all members of a community having particular roles based on individual qualities.

During the 20th century, a shift took place towards large, long-stay asylums for people with intellectual disabilities. Later, these were designated as hospitals, and in the UK came under the umbrella of the National Health Service.[1] As a result, people with intellectual disabilities experienced an increase in segregation and isolation, and a decrease in meaningful roles and activities, and with it, more stigmatization. Not only this, but, appallingly, the concept of eugenics was also internationally popular in the early 20th century.

In the 1980s and 90s, there was growing concern about people's experiences of long-stay institutions, leading to the shift towards de-institutionalization and normalization (Wolfensberger et al., 1972). With this came the concept of 'care in the community' (Audit Commission, 1986), which focused on people's rights to live in ordinary houses on ordinary streets. While this brought benefits for many (but not all), it has not been the end of societal

---

[1]   The National Health Service (NHS) was founded in 1948 and was set up to provide everyone in the UK with healthcare based on their needs and not their ability to pay. The NHS is a service which is 'free' at the point of access to individuals living in the United Kingdom (funded by general taxation and National Insurance payments by working people).

challenges for people with intellectual disabilities. Living in an ordinary house in a village or town is not the same as being meaningfully connected to the community among whom one is living. The results in achieving such connections have been mixed.

In addition, some people with intellectual disabilities remain in hospital because they have other difficulties in respect of 'behaviours that challenge' and/or mental health struggles. Certainly, in the UK, some people continue to find themselves admitted to hospital and stuck there for long periods. This often happens when support providers report that they can no longer support the person. This is partly a factor of the person's difficulties at the time, but it can also be related to the provider's skill level, staff support, staffing levels, staff morale and the appropriateness of placements (linked to a lack of available options).

In recent years in the UK there has been a strong national agenda to reduce unnecessary hospital admissions and improve community support, known as Transforming Care (Department of Health, 2012). This was triggered by scandals such as the 2012 Winterbourne View hospital investigation. *Panaroma*, a British investigative television programme, exposed abuse and criminal acts of assault by supporters on people with intellectual disabilities detained under the Mental Health Act. Much work has been done since to try to ensure that people are not required to stay in hospitals far from their home areas. However, barriers continue to exist in terms of finding support agencies who are highly skilled at supporting people with the most complex needs. There remains a long way to go to achieve the now much delayed objectives of the Transforming Care agenda (DHSC, 2012).

Societal norms and attitudes run deep and often below the conscious level, particularly in our use of language. It is worth remembering that several derogatory terms still in common use have origins in describing people with intellectual disabilities, which sheds light on some of these cultural biases. Many are considered highly offensive. Some words are so embedded in our day-to-day speech that they are widely used and accepted by many (e.g. the words 'idiot' and 'stupid' or referring to someone as 'simple'). The use of pejorative language is much less accepted in relation to other characteristics such as race, gender or sexuality. This highlights the position that people with intellectual disabilities still have in society.

On a more positive note, in recent years there has been significant societal focus on increasing inclusion and addressing discrimination against minoritized people and groups, including intellectual diversity, and there has been a much greater focus on neurodiversity, such as autism and ADHD. There are, additionally, some positive signs of change for people with intellectual disabilities, with invaluable support and championing from family members, paid supporters, charities, organizations and advocates. This is still getting nowhere near the publicity and recognition that neurodiverse conditions such as ADHD and autism do, so there is still much work to be done.

Health inequalities for people with intellectual disabilities

Despite seemingly positive steps to address health inequalities, it is worrying that people with intellectual disabilities continue to die at a far younger age than people without intellectual disabilities. A growing body of evidence suggests that people with intellectual disabilities experience a greater number of health conditions than the wider population, including epilepsy, obesity, coronary heart disease, malnutrition, constipation, mental health problems, increased risk of cancer, diabetes, oral health issues, dementia and respiratory conditions (Mencap, n.d.).

Health difficulties may be exacerbated for people with intellectual disabilities by barriers to accessing good-quality healthcare. These include lack of accessible transport links and confidence in travelling to medical appointments, diagnostic overshadowing (attribution of health conditions to intellectual disability), communication difficulties, limited understanding of intellectual disabilities by a person's support network or health professionals, failure by services to implement necessary reasonable adjustments to support understanding of health conditions or ways to nurture quality of life, a limited support network and social isolation.

The LeDeR (Learning Disability Mortality Review) programme has been set up in the UK (NHS England, 2021). This is a service improvement programme to investigate factors associated with the deaths of people with intellectual disabilities. These deaths are often premature. A Confidential Inquiry by Heslop et al. (2013) found that nearly 25 percent of people with intellectual disabilities were younger than 50 years when they died, and the median age of death of male individuals with intellectual disabilities was 13 years younger than the median age at death of male individuals in the general population of England and Wales, and 20 years younger for females. The 2022 LeDeR mortality review found that there had been 'gentle but continuous improvement' in the median age of death for people with a learning disability in 2022. In 2018, the median age of death for adults with a learning disability was 61.8 years but has since risen to 62.9 in 2022. A drop was also found in the number of avoidable deaths since 2021 – 42 percent of deaths were deemed 'avoidable' for people with a learning disability in 2022 compared to 50 percent in 2021. Whilst this is encouraging, there is still a long way to go.

Promisingly, some positive steps have been taken to address such stark inequalities. These include the implementation of health-promotion initiatives such as annual health checks, flu immunization and cancer screening, as well as effective and meaningful reasonable adjustments such as provision of easy-read information, avoidance of medical jargon and longer appointment times. However, it is still crucial to recognize that, when working with people with intellectual disabilities, their health and their healthcare may be poorer than the general population, and health issues must be considered via biopsychosocial formulations (Allez et al., 2023).

The downsides of being cared for

The late American psychologist Herb Lovett wrote powerfully about the rights of people with intellectual disabilities in the 1980s and 1990s (e.g. Lovett, 1996). Whilst there have undoubtedly been huge changes in societal attitudes in the intervening years, relevant gems remain to be found in Lovett's writings, particularly with regard to equality and power. Lovett reflected on some of the difficult truths about the drawbacks of receiving care and support from others, often in terms of control of one's own life and sometimes in terms of dignity. Lovett also noted that the labels given to people by health services can get in the way of seeing the person. A gap can develop between what we (intuitively) know and what we (professionals) do. Of particular note is Lovett's view that 'people whose behaviour is difficult are not people to be fixed so much as freedom fighters – the most vigorous critics of our attempts at service' (Lovett, 1996, p.6). Powerfully, Lovett also posits that the most extreme behaviour often comes from not feeling listened to.

Services that aim to support and help the person can in fact sometimes locate the problem within the individual. In other words, there is a tendency to attribute the reasons for a person's difficulties to deficits within that person rather than considering the wider contextual factors that may be causing or exacerbating their difficulties. Sometimes, the wider system fails to view a person's behaviours from a functional perspective. Supporters' responses become perpetuating rather than protective factors. For example, supporters may become exasperated and adopt a more punitive parental response to a person's risky behaviours (such as self-harming). They may lack empathy for behaviour that arises from a need for care and support, driving the person further towards the behaviour. People can become 'othered' and common humanity becomes forgotten about (Lovett, 1996).

Despite the great work of many in the field, there is a long way to go before people with intellectual disabilities are truly and practically treated as equal members of society with the same needs as anyone else.

The consequences of feeling unheard

Feeling unheard and not listened to can lead to expressions of emotion that may be misinterpreted by services and labelled as 'challenging behaviour'. This can result in referrals to specialist services for support to 'fix' the behaviour. Over many years, the term 'challenging behaviour' has morphed from a description of the responsibilities of services to understand and meet needs, to a pseudodiagnostic label (i.e. something that a person 'has'). This can result in further stigmatization and exclusion from society. People whose behaviours present the greatest challenges for services are sometimes moved to hospital or residential settings many miles from their home and family due to a lack of adequate local support.

Challenging behaviour has typically been defined in the following way:

> Behaviour can be described as challenging when it is of such an intensity, frequency, or duration as to threaten the quality of life and/or the physical safety of the individual or others and it is likely to lead to responses that are restrictive, aversive or result in exclusion. (Royal College of Psychiatrists et al., 2007, p.10).

Recently, the term has rightly evolved to move away from a description of the problem as being within the person, towards describing the behaviour as a challenge to services that attempt to provide support. Nowadays, the preferred term is 'behaviours that may challenge'. This recognizes that whether something is challenging or not depends on the context and perception of others, rather than this being something fixed and 'within' the person. Other people prefer to refer to 'distress behaviours'. This shift in language and ideology encourages services and professionals to explore the unmet needs that underlie behavioural presentations. It aims to find effective, holistic and person-centred ways of understanding and supporting individuals with intellectual disabilities.

The way language is used is certainly important and will be explored later in this book.

Scope to make mistakes

One of the ways in which people with intellectual disabilities may be treated differently is in how much tolerance is shown when mistakes are made. Making mistakes is typically the privilege of those in majority (non-excluded) groups. But for people with intellectual disabilities, a difficulty or failure may be seen as the person being unable to do something, rather than a sign that they may benefit from further opportunities, skill development or encouragement. This may result in their being afforded fewer opportunities to work through difficulties, which may lead to a cycle of placement breakdown and frequent placement moves.

Supporters can sometimes (understandably) be anxious about the potential of risk of harm to the person. This creates a discrepancy between what the person with an intellectual disability wants to do, and what the supporter believes is in their best interests to keep them safe. The desire to keep someone 'safe' can inadvertently reduce the person's opportunities to have normal, everyday experiences.

As a slight, but hopefully useful, aside, we recommend the reader to refer to the 'Keeping Me Safe and Well' resource (Greenhill & Whitehead, 2010). This is a human-rights based, positive risk-taking tool that we have found helpful in encouraging supporters to keep the person central and to help ensure supporters are not overly risk averse.

Context is key

Understanding the contextual factors underpinning the presentation of a person with intellectual disabilities is key to a thorough assessment and subsequent formulation of the wider picture. The wider picture considers all aspects of individual circumstances. We are all shaped by our experiences and wider contexts. This can be even more fundamental to appreciate for people with intellectual disabilities. This is a population who may not be able to volunteer this type of important information, and whose history may be lost due to moving homes and information not being transferred with them. Sometimes, processes and policies around data retention within public services can make historical information difficult or impossible to gather. We must understand someone's experiences, because missing key aspects of the picture can lead to less effective/appropriate therapeutic interventions.

The social model of disability emerged in the 1970s, developed by disabled people. This social model posits that people have impairments rather than disabilities; and that oppression and exclusion of, and discrimination against, people with such impairments are caused by society as opposed to being situated within the person (Inclusion London, 2015). In our work, we should consider ways in which difficulties can be considered contextually, not just in terms of difficulties that a person 'has'. This fits very well with a theoretical philosophy underpinning ACT known as 'functional contextualism', which we will go on to describe in Chapter 2.

Trauma and ACEs

A raft of factors have the potential to influence human presentation. We know that Adverse Childhood Events (ACEs) which include types of childhood abuse, neglect and household dysfunction, are linked to later difficulties and negative outcomes (Felitti et al., 1998).

ACEs are more common for people with disabilities, including intellectual disabilities (Reichman et al., 2018). Studies have shown that both children and adults with intellectual disabilities are more likely to experience traumatic events (Dion et al., 2018; Nixon et al., 2017), yet in practice trauma is an underrecognized issue for this population. Given this, their resilience is striking: we frequently encounter individuals who have suffered horrific experiences and yet still manage to find the good in others and develop positive and trusting relationships.

Of course, some people do require trauma intervention, direct and/or indirect. In the UK, NICE (the National Institute for Health and Care Excellence) guidance currently recommends two types of therapies: trauma-focused cognitive behavioural therapy (CBT) and Eye Movement Desensitization Reprocessing (EMDR) as the therapeutic approaches to trauma (NICE, 2018). ACT is increasingly used, either as a standalone alternative or as an adjunct to CBT/EMDR. There is emerging research evidence for the use of ACT for trauma presentations (Pohar & Argáez, 2017; Simoes & Silva, 2021).

Any suitability assessment for ACT intervention should involve the exploration of possible past ACEs/later traumas, and their impact on current functioning. This can be challenging, because trauma symptoms can manifest differently and can be difficult for people with intellectual disabilities to identify and report. Fortunately, some established assessment tools for identifying trauma symptoms in someone with an intellectual disability now exist, for example, the LANTS (Lancaster and Northgate Trauma Scales: Wigham, Hatton & Taylor, 2021) or the IES-LD (Impact of Event Scale for People with Learning Disabilities: Hall, Jobson & Langdon, 2014). These lack normative data[2] but nonetheless are very useful tools to help practitioners to be alert to the possibility of trauma forming a part of the presenting picture.

It is important not to assume that the experience of traumatic events requires intervention. Some people, particularly those with good social networks, active coping skills, good self-care, optimism and cognitive flexibility are resilient despite their experiences (Iacoviello & Charney, 2014).

---

2   Normative data is data from a reference population (typically the general population) that establishes a baseline distribution for a score or measurement to allow comparison (Campbell, 2013). In this case, we are referring to a lack of an average score or a score that indicates a threshold or cut-off has been reached that indicates clinical concern.

That said, sometimes what appears to be resilience is in fact the masking and suppression of difficulties, which therefore requires careful assessment. Masking refers to someone's ability to hide their difficulties in order to fit in; and whilst the term is most often used in relation to autistic people, in our experience, masking is also used by many people with ID. However, we wish to highlight that someone who does not show resilience is not weak or lacking in any way: rather, they have not had the good fortune to be afforded the factors that foster resilience.

As we will go on to discuss in later chapters, factors positively influencing resilience can all be addressed through use of the ACT model through the building up of full, values-based lives.

Intersectionality

In the wider context of a person's life, it is important to consider other marginalized aspects of the person in addition to the intellectual disability. The person may also be from an ethnic minority background, identify as gay, bisexual, transgender (or any other form of LGBT+ identity), or be from a minority religious background (Dunlop & Lea, 2023).

Different identities or forms of marginalization can interact and result in a unique experience of the world for the person, known as *intersectionality*. It will be important to be curious about and honour the person's unique perspectives and experiences in relation to intersectionality, even if they are not always able to articulate these due to cognitive and language difficulties. For example, consider the person's demographics and how these are likely to feed into the overall picture.

People whose identities are minoritized are also at risk of minority stress, due to their needs and views differing from dominant mainstream narratives. People from majority groups may have less experience and understanding of minority perspectives. Practitioners working with people with intellectual disabilities who are members of other minoritized groups should consider the interplay of these different layers of identities. As practitioners we should also consider our own blind spots and potential areas of bias, for example through the use of supervision and further study.

CASE STUDY: Joel

Joel, a 25-year-old man, presented with difficulties with alcohol and drugs and low mood. Joel had a mild intellectual disability, and likely (but as yet undiagnosed) neurodiversity. Joel grew up in an area of low socioeconomic status. He was White Eastern-European and a gay man. Joel often presented as seemingly hostile and defensive. He frequently engaged in risky sexual behaviours and drug-taking. This put him into contact with the criminal justice system.

Joel did not refer to any contextual factors within sessions, yet factors such as limited finances, being from a minority ethnic background and sexual orientation, as well as experiencing historical trauma and stigmatization, all undoubtedly were relevant. They had a significant impact upon his relationships with others, sense of identity and empowerment. Raising this as a possibility to Joel and generating discussion was validating for him and enabled his difficulties to be placed within context. This allowed the therapeutic relationship to develop and thus reduced Joel's defensiveness. This, in turn, enabled him to make positive changes alongside the practitioner, working with supporters, to make appropriate reasonable adjustments and address systemic barriers such as finances and access to local social and support groups.

Supporters' attributions

Attribution theory (Heider, 1958) focuses on an individual's perception of the cause of events and behaviours. Attributions about why a person's behaviour is 'challenging' will influence the ways in which a supporter responds, affecting the support provided (Griffith & Hastings, 2014). Every paid supporter has their own personal story, and their own unique reasons for choosing to work within a support work setting. Each supporter brings along their own attitudes, beliefs and style. These inevitably shape the conscious and subconscious ways in which support is provided. Lack of resources and natural human emotions such as stress, fatigue and frustration can challenge a supporter's resilience, making it harder to cope with certain aspects of the role, which may be emotionally loaded due their own personal histories. Evidence suggests that supporters' direct experience of behaviours that challenge can lead to negative emotional reactions and poor psychological wellbeing, such as burnout, emotional exhaustion and depersonalization (Skirrow & Hatton, 2007). Opportunities for reflective support within a safe, supportive and confidential space are of utmost importance. This allows scope for attributions to be safely explored and challenged so that supporters feel equipped in their role.

Unfortunately, not all supporters have this opportunity. While some can be highly attuned to the person they support, high stress levels and limited training and support can lead to interactions between person and supporter that are unhelpful, and at its most extreme, neglectful or abusive.

Empowerment and resilience

Despite the challenges faced by many people with intellectual disabilities, there are also numerous examples of real progress: for example, the development of self-advocacy groups, and experts-by-experience being meaningfully involved in recruitment and co-production of the development of health and social care services.

There are also numerous examples of personal achievements that have entered public awareness. In the UK, the TV presenter and author George Webster has spoken and written about his experiences as a person with Down's syndrome. His book aimed at children with developmental differences has some inspiring quotes, including the following: 'Each one of us is different, just like pebbles at the seaside. Together we make a bigger splash and spread our glow far and wide' (Webster, 2023, p.13). In the UK, we are witnessing an increase in people with intellectual disabilities in the media, including in acting roles and even in news reporting, something that once would have been thought impossible.

Whilst in the UK, it is incredibly disappointing that reviews of The Transforming Care agenda have found that targets around reducing hospital admissions have not been met, and evidence of high use of restraint in care settings has emerged, we have witnessed a change within community services. There is an increase in scrutiny of hospital admissions and the implementation of local risk registers and Community and Treatment Reviews, which are regular reviews of a person's care either when at risk of hospital admission or in hospital, aimed at preventing, or minimizing the length of, admission.

Psychological approaches

We have highlighted the inequity and injustice that has historically been, and still continues to be, experienced by people with intellectual disabilities, resulting in a high prevalence of psychological distress. This begs the question: How do we support people with intellectual disabilities with their psychological wellbeing?

There was a time when the idea of offering psychological therapies to people with intellectual disabilities was seen as radical, and behaviourism was the most commonly used approach. Behavioural approaches can still very much be helpful today: for example, avoiding negative or positive reinforcement, or consideration of concepts such as intermittent reinforcement, differential reinforcement, fading out or flooding. However, historically, influenced by how people with intellectual disabilities were seen in society, such methods could sometimes lack ethical standards and at their worst involved (which seems incredible now), using punitive methods, including cold showers or spraying lemon juice in people's eyes.

An important milestone was in 1993, when Mike Bender highlighted what he described as 'therapeutic disdain' among mental health professionals when working with people with intellectual disabilities. This referred to the tendency to exclude people from therapy due to the view that they would be unable to access it effectively. This tendency has perhaps not completely been eradicated, since Mills et al.'s (2023) study showed that people with intellectual disabilities and mental health problems were most likely to be provided Positive Behavioural Support (PBS: Carr et al., 1999), a popular framework in the UK based on applied behavioural analysis, but not specific psychological therapies. Of course, there are many circumstances where a behavioural approach may be entirely the correct one. However, there is often scope to consider what kind of direct skills and therapeutic work may also be beneficial for the person.

Despite the higher prevalence rates of mental health difficulties among people with intellectual disabilities in comparison to the general population, robust empirical evidence regarding the clinical effectiveness of therapeutic interventions remains limited (Osugo & Cooper, 2016). Whilst the evidence base for psychological therapies remains emergent, in practice it is now common for adapted talking therapies to be provided by services. A wide range of approaches have been used: for example, psychodynamic therapy (Beail et al., 2005), cognitive behavioural therapy (e.g. Willner, 2009; Willner, Rose & Jahoda, 2014), Behavioural Activation for Depression (Jahoda et al., 2024) and EMDR (Barrowcliff & Evans, 2015).

Difficulties with communication and understanding that are associated with people with intellectual disabilities may affect meaningful engagement with traditional therapeutic approaches (Chinn et al., 2014). To overcome these problems, emerging evidence suggests that modification of standard psychological interventions may enhance accessibility of mainstream approaches (Osugo & Cooper, 2016). Sturmey (2004) argued that much of the change seen in the lives of people with intellectual disabilities as a result of psychological therapies is related to the underpinning behavioural components. For example, within Sturmey's selective review of cognitive therapy for people with intellectual disabilities, results indicated that many interventions such as anger management were in fact packages that included many behavioural interventions such as relaxation and social-skills training, alongside some cognitive methods such as cognitive restructuring.

This poses the question as to whether change was underpinned by cognitive aspects of therapy versus the implicit behavioural approach. However, CBT can be adapted to maximize the likelihood of people with intellectual disabilities benefiting from both its behavioural and cognitive elements (Willner, 2009). We know that the meta-ability required to identify and alter one's response to cognitions is challenging for many people. However, it is indeed possible for some people to benefit from cognitive interventions, albeit often with some prior preparatory and educative work, which we discuss in more depth in the following chapters.

Finally, we should remember that there is well-established research suggesting that in fact the therapeutic relationship is the key determining factor for therapy outcomes (Keijsers, Schaap & Hoogduin, 2000). There is no reason to suggest that this is any different for people with intellectual disabilities. When using ACT, as with any therapy, we must pay attention to building rapport and remembering principles of unconditional positive regard, empathy and congruence, pioneered by Carl Rogers (1959, cited in Bozarth, 2007). When working therapeutically with people who have often experienced a lifetime of disempowerment and many experiences of being let down and 'othered', this is all the more important. We implore you to use the ACT practices and techniques judiciously, always keeping the relational elements of therapy in mind.

SUMMARY

+ There are some contextual and historical factors that should be kept in mind when formulating and working with people with intellectual disabilities, including this population's experience of segregation, abuse and a lack of control over their own lives.

+ The most significant change in the UK in recent decades has been the move to community-based provision and the increased scrutiny of these settings, as well as hospital provision. We recognize that the move to community-based care has not yet resulted in people with intellectual disabilities living normal and equal lives.

+ ACT practitioners must consider contextual factors when formulating and adapting ACT to people with intellectual disabilities, particularly being mindful of issues of disempowerment and trauma.

+ People with intellectual disabilities continue to face stigma, inappropriate practices and a lack of services. However, therapeutic support is now a viable option, representing a positive change in the mindset of those designing and delivering services.

Chapter 2

WHAT IS ACCEPTANCE AND COMMITMENT THERAPY AND WHY USE IT?

In this chapter a case is built for ACT as a relevant and powerful therapeutic approach. We begin with a brief description of what ACT is and provide an outline of the key features of mainstream (non-adapted) ACT as a model. We then discuss why ACT can be useful when working with people with intellectual disabilities. At the end of this chapter, there is a list of introductory ACT reading materials, which we recommend to enhance the experience of using this book.

The origins of ACT

Recent developments in psychological therapy have led to the emergence of a modern generation of behavioural therapies, including Acceptance and Commitment Therapy (ACT). This is sometimes described as a 'third wave' behavioural therapy. The first wave (mostly) had a traditional focus on observable behaviours rather than thoughts or emotions. The second wave incorporates Beck's cognitive therapy (Beck, 1976), bringing in thoughts as a legitimate focus for interventions. Third-wave approaches typically have a broader focus on achieving better quality of life, rather than a primary focus on reduction of symptoms, and incorporate mindfulness and acceptance-oriented features. Other third-wave approaches include Dialectical Behaviour Therapy (Linehan, 1993), Mindfulness Based Cognitive Therapy (Segal, Williams & Teasdale, 2012), and (arguably) Compassion Focused Therapy (Gilbert, 2000).

ACT itself was developed by Professor Steven Hayes and his colleagues Kelly Wilson and Kirk Strosahl (Hayes, Strosahl & Wilson, 1999). It was later built upon by others, including Robin Walser, Louise Hayes, and Russ

Harris. Steven Hayes has described the early ACT concepts as incorporating a range of sources. Hayes has a background in radical behaviourism, having worked with and been inspired by giants in the field of behaviourism, including B.F. Skinner. Hayes saw a need to incorporate a person's internal experiences (thoughts, emotions, sensations). Hayes and colleagues also had concerns that the emerging cognitive behavioural therapies seemed to lack a coherent theory of psychological wellbeing that was linked to the evidence at the time. Hayes argued that second-wave behavioural therapies seemed to be more of a pragmatic melding of traditional behaviourism and a focus on cognitions, without a sound theoretical underpinning that encompassed both aspects. Hayes and others also questioned the science behind the focus on challenging and changing thought patterns, which represented a central feature of early CBT models (Zettle & Rains, 1989; Zettle, Rains & Hayes, 2011). He also noted that his own personal history of struggling with a panic disorder had shown him first-hand both the futility of trying to suppress and ignore difficult thoughts and emotions, and the utility of approaches that focus on making room for and accepting emotional responses. Having an earlier history of living in communes and being exposed to Eastern philosophies in the 1960s allowed Hayes to draw upon aspects of meditation and mindfulness principles, which were subsequently incorporated into ACT. Despite the inclusion of these aspects, ACT focuses on techniques that could be used in day-to-day situations and would be acceptable to people who may not wish to engage in frequent prolonged meditation practices.

Intellectual disability practitioners are usually very familiar with the behavioural approaches and traditions from which ACT has developed. What may be less well known is that ACT has developed from a particular branch of behaviourism known as functional contextualism (Biglan & Hayes, 1996) and incorporates an understanding of human language drawing from Relational Frame Theory (RFT: Barnes-Holmes et al., 2001).

An excellent summary of both theories is provided by Hayes (2004). It is important to include the warning that this material has some quite complex and technical theoretical underpinnings. Still, a working understanding of these principles can further enhance one's work as an ACT practitioner.

Functional contextualism

In the most basic terms, a functional contextual perspective is based on assumptions that all behaviour occurs within particular contexts and not in isolation (i.e. not emerging entirely as something within the individual). All behaviour has meaning, serves a function, fulfils unmet physical or emotional needs, and is not random.

From a functional contextual point of view, there is no ultimate truth, only pragmatic truth. In other words, a person's actions are not inherently right or wrong; it depends upon the situation (context) and the function it has. In ACT, this links to a concept described as 'workability'. Workability is less about whether a belief, idea or rule is 'true' or 'false' but about how well it serves a person in living their life according to what matters to them. If it does, it can be described as workable; but if it prevents or interferes with progress towards a values-based goal, then it can be described as unworkable.

Within the ACT model, the term 'behaviour' encompasses anything the individual does. This includes internal events, such as thoughts or memories, as well as external events, such as actions. The functional analysis of behaviours is the 'bread and butter' of most practitioners working with people with intellectual disabilities and can be defined as 'a method for understanding the causes and consequences of behaviour and its relationship to particular stimuli, and the function of the behaviour' (National Collaborating Centre for Mental Health, 2015).

Within an applied behavioural analysis framework, functions of behaviours can be broadly categorized into four key functions:

- escape/avoidance
- tangible
- social attention
- sensory.

While it might be seen as reductive to consider behaviours in terms of four key functions, the idea that behaviours have a function is a useful focus within ACT, as it connects directly with the concept of workability: determining whether a behaviour is effective in helping a person live a meaningful life. However, as practitioners, we would also combine looking at behaviours alongside richer individual formulations.

Sadly, there has historically been too great an emphasis on eliminating behaviours displayed by a person with an intellectual disability, rather than establishing the function and subsequently more workable alternatives to the behaviour (if current behaviours are deemed not workable). The development and proliferation of the behavioural model 'positive behaviour support' (PBS: Allen et al., 2005), underpinned by the functional analysis of behaviours, has served to shift this emphasis. In Chapter 10 we describe how ACT can be used when developing PBS plans.

Relational Frame Theory

Relational Frame Theory focuses on human language development, and the process of learning verbal 'rules'. Language involves learning to respond to the relations between stimuli – for example, the relation between words and objects (a particular object is called a *cup*), or between and among words (e.g. *hot* is the opposite of *cold*, a *dollar* is worth more than a *dime*). This process allows people to organize, predict and control how consequences are obtained in relation to the context. This way, you can anticipate future situations without having experienced them. This is known as creating verbal rules.

This ability to create relationships in language is a double-edged sword, since humans are equally able to form negative judgements of themselves or others, based on imagined or feared scenarios, or negative past experiences. Research has shown that whilst animal behaviours are influenced by actual events ('contingencies') in their environment, humans tend to continue to apply verbal rules once formed. This means that we are sometimes less attuned to our environments, and can be overly focused on our own thoughts, beliefs and rules. Paradoxically, our clever brains with their amazing language skills can actually get in the way of learning from experiences. They keep us stuck in a vicious cycle of psychological suffering, repeatedly drawing upon ineffective strategies for change. Relational frame theorists argue that, once formed, verbal rules cannot be erased, only added to.

However, the *relationship* a person has with their thoughts can make a big difference: for example, whether a person is caught up and driven by thoughts that they are unlovable, or whether they can find ways to reduce the impact of such thoughts and continue doing the things they want to be doing.

What ACT aims to do

Professor Steven Hayes defines ACT as

> a unique, empirically based psychological intervention that uses acceptance and mindfulness strategies, together with commitment and behaviour change strategies, to increase psychological flexibility. Psychological flexibility means contacting the present moment fully as a conscious human being, and based on what the situation affords, changing or persisting in behaviour in the service of chosen values. (Association for Contextual Behavioral Science, n.d.)

From an ACT perspective, living lives as consistent with one's values as possible and doing what matters (to the person) is key to good mental health and quality of life. If we shut down our lives out of fear or depression, we suffer more. If we are living lives based on the perceived values of others, or without a clear idea about what our own values are, we neglect ourselves and risk living a life lacking in fulfilment.

If we cannot experience the present moment, whether that moment is savouring or suffering, we lose opportunities for joy and/or suppress difficult emotions. Suppressed emotions build up and often find their outlets in unhelpful or more extreme ways (e.g. panic attacks or anger). It is human nature to defend against difficult realities and experiences in a whole range of ways, whether this is rationalizing, emotional numbing via alcohol, drugs, sex or self-harm, or being defensive or hostile – the list goes on. Such efforts inevitably lead to further suffering.

ACT therefore aims for openness to experience, *just as it is* – whether this be to psychological distress, feeling vulnerable and taking managed risks towards what matters, or self-permission to feel joy. The overall aim of ACT is to increase psychological flexibility.

Psychological flexibility

Psychological flexibility can be defined as:

> contacting the present moment as a conscious human being, fully and without needless defence – as it is and not what it says it is – and persisting with or changing a behaviour in the service of chosen values. (Hayes, Strosahl & Wilson, 2011, p.96)

In straightforward terms, this means that the focus of ACT interventions is to support people in making choices to move towards what really matters, whilst embracing the inevitable difficulties associated with action which may not always feel like the safest, easiest or most straightforward option.

ACT is a process-based therapy; in other words, there is a focus upon what we know about processes that can be effective in therapy based on a biopsychosocial formulation as opposed to a prescriptive manual based on a diagnosis. Rather, ACT developers have identified some of the most common factors or processes that impact upon psychological wellbeing, and on their flipside, psychological distress. These can and should be focused on in a flexibly tailored way, depending on individual need.

The Hexaflex

The 'Hexaflex' (Figure 2.1) outlines the six core therapeutic processes in ACT: Acceptance, Defusion, Contact with the Present Moment, Self-as-Context, Values, and Committed Action.

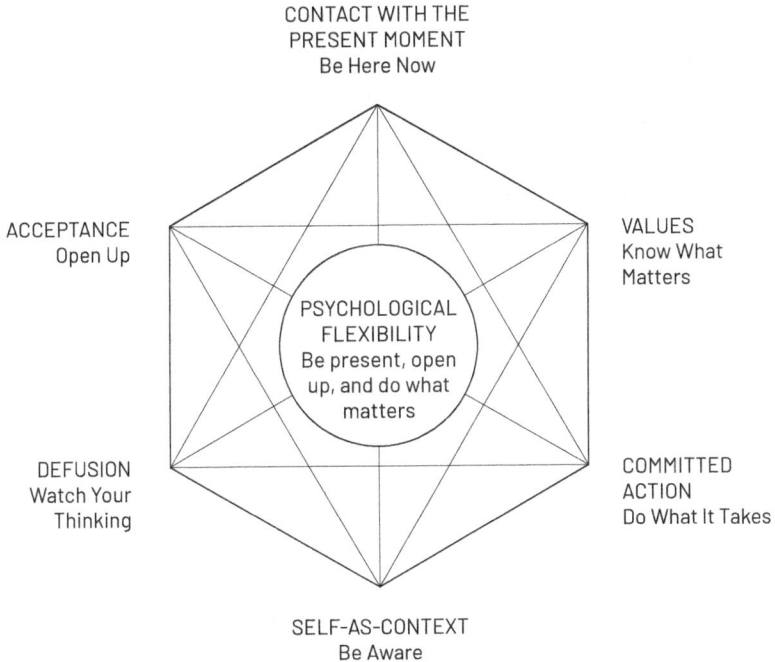

CONTACT WITH THE
PRESENT MOMENT
Be Here Now

ACCEPTANCE
Open Up

VALUES
Know What
Matters

PSYCHOLOGICAL
FLEXIBILITY
Be present, open
up, and do what
matters

DEFUSION
Watch Your
Thinking

COMMITTED
ACTION
Do What It Takes

SELF-AS-CONTEXT
Be Aware

Figure 2.1 *The Hexaflex (Hayes, Strosahl & Wilson, 2011)*

Acceptance (Open Up)

Acceptance approaches focus upon the willingness to open up to difficult thoughts, feelings and memories: allowing them to be, just as they are. By making room for unpleasant or unwanted psychological experiences, the struggle becomes less, and we make space for them to be. This does not mean having to like or actively seek difficult psychological experiences. The aim is simply to make space for their existence, dropping the ongoing battle to eradicate them completely. Nor does it mean accepting abusive or unjust experiences. This is a highly important distinction when the contexts of the lives of people with intellectual disabilities are considered.

The emphasis is on a differentiation between those situations that cannot be changed (requiring acceptance) and those that can be improved through effective action (which links to the commitment domains).

Defusion (Watch Your Thinking)

Defusion involves training our minds to consciously 'step back' and untangle ourselves from our internal cognitive processes, such as thoughts, images and memories. Using Defusion skills, thoughts, memories and images are allowed to come and go as they please. The aim here is to 'watch them' come and go, just like trains passing through a station, clouds floating across the sky or leaves on a stream. The struggle to push thoughts away or to alter them is let go – the aim is to hold them lightly, let them be, view them from a distance and notice them for exactly what they are.

Contact with the Present Moment (Be Here Now)

This domain involves skills to improve a person's ability to pay attention to what is actually occurring in the here and now, as opposed to being preoccupied with the past or worried about the future. The present-moment aspects of ACT are about building skills to enable a person to pay attention to what is happening to them at any given moment. When we are more present, whether this be to our surroundings and/or our inner experiences, we are more able to live life fully and experience it as it actually is.

Self-as-Context (Be Aware)

Self-as-Context encourages a focus on the 'observing self', the aspect of ourselves that has been ever present. Despite life changes, role changes, ageing and growth, the part of us that 'observes' has been there all along. This aspect of the Hexaflex encourages us to zoom in on this observing process and recognize that there are two distinct elements to the mind. This is perhaps one of the most abstract elements of ACT, but it can still be used with people with intellectual disabilities in a simplified form (see Chapter 3).

Values (Know What Matters)

Values are the crux of the ACT model. Different from goals, values are the qualities that truly matter to us, deep down. Values are never 'achieved' or 'completed' but instead offer a compass direction for individuals to choose to move towards at all times, despite life's challenges. A clear grasp of values is essential to moving towards a meaningful life. They are compass points to guide valued direction in life, towards the things that truly matter in our hearts.

Committed Action (Do What It Takes)

This involves a clear and conscious effort to move towards valued aspects of life. Guided by a compass direction of values, the things that truly matter, individuals are encouraged to make a choice to catch the things that matter and move towards those, despite difficult or unpleasant emotions, thoughts or sensations that may arise.

ACT and psychological flexibility

A central tenet of the ACT model is that psychological inflexibility, and therefore psychological suffering, arises from difficulties in the six domains within Figure 2.1. Put simply, if we are not living in the here and now, not doing what matters to us, and we are 'fused with' our difficult thoughts and feelings or resistant to difficult experiences, our lives become less fulfilling. Repeated experiential avoidance (the avoidance of unwanted experiences) and a focus on getting rid of, or trying in a myriad of ways to push away, troubling thoughts and emotions can result in a narrowing of one's life. Subsequently, this can have a seemingly paradoxical negative impact upon mental health and overall wellbeing.

An ACT intervention, therefore, focuses on reducing rigidity in the six Hexaflex domains to allow individuals to become more attuned to what matters and what works, rather than a narrow focus on reduction of notable symptoms. Such an approach can be extremely useful for many people with intellectual disabilities who can struggle with inflexibility of thinking and difficulty in learning from experiences, as well as useful to their supporters who may experience high levels of work-related stress and burnout (Leoni et al., 2016; Noone & Hastings, 2009) and whose support is often vital to the person with intellectual disability.

Formulating using the ACT model

Formulation is an important aspect of any therapeutic approach. Defined as 'a process of ongoing collaborative sense-making' (Harper & Moss, 2003), formulation can take a multitude of formats according to the model or models being used. It can also be described as a personal story or narrative that has been collaboratively and dynamically developed (Johnstone and Dallos, 2006), or as a 'summary/integration of a broad range of biopsychosocial causal factors based on personal meaning and collaboratively constructed' (Division of Clinical Psychology, 2011).

Five Ps formulation

When using ACT, there are various ways in which to formulate. The 'Five Ps' model (Macneil et al., 2012) is a broad model that takes into consideration presenting problems, predisposing factors, perpetuating factors, protective factors and precipitating factors. This can be useful especially where you have not yet specified which therapeutic approach you are using, or where you wish to ensure you have a broader formulation. We often use the Five Ps model in clinical practice, particularly in the early stages of piecing together a person's history and current situation.

The Five Ps model offers a thorough means of capturing information from a variety of sources and individuals involved with someone. An example template of the Five Ps formulation model developed by one of the authors is included below (Figure 2.2a), This is often completed collaboratively during early therapy sessions alongside the individual (and support team where appropriate) (Figure 2.2b). It is a useful tool to focus sessions that take place via video/teleconferencing, a practice that has become more common following on from the Covid-19 pandemic. The focus on a shared document on-screen has encouraged genuine collaborative formulation.

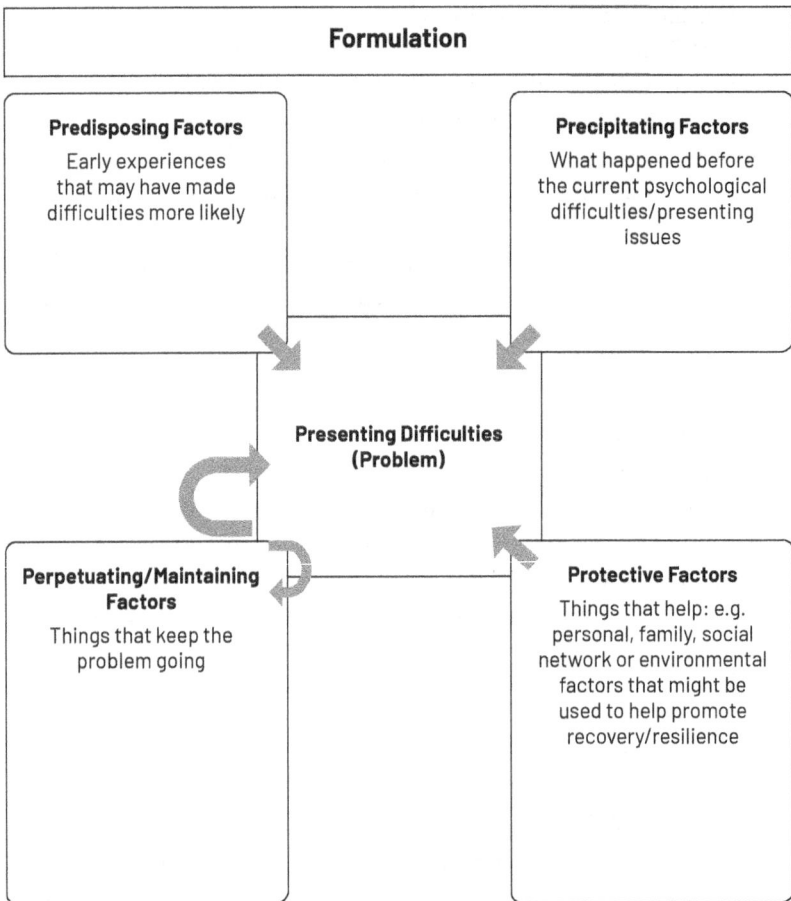

Formulation

Predisposing Factors
Early experiences that may have made difficulties more likely

Precipitating Factors
What happened before the current psychological difficulties/presenting issues

Presenting Difficulties (Problem)

Perpetuating/Maintaining Factors
Things that keep the problem going

Protective Factors
Things that help: e.g. personal, family, social network or environmental factors that might be used to help promote recovery/resilience

Figure 2.2a The Five Ps formulation model

Formulation

Values: Family, health and fitness, outdoor pursuits, loyalty, respect, kindness.

Predisposing Factors

Early experiences that may have made difficulties more likely

Intellectual disability

Autism

Difficult early attachment experiences – taken into care aged 2

Maternal mental health difficulties, and substance use during pregnancy

Precipitating Factors

What happened before the current psychological difficulties/presenting issues

Placement moves throughout life

Bereavement, loss of two grandparents within one year

Placement breakdown

Presenting Difficulties (Problem)

Substance use (alcohol and drugs)

Aggression towards staff and peers

Recent incarceration due to burglary

Perpetuating/Maintaining Factors

Things that keep the problem going

Lack of stable base, place to call home

Isolation, boredom, lack of meaningful occupation – minimal sense of purpose in life; no reason to get up in the morning

Rumination about events from the past and worries about potential future eventualities

Protective Factors

Things that help: e.g. personal, family, social network or environmental factors that might be used to help promote recovery/resilience

An emphasis on values-based ventures at the heart of support

Regular use of and practice of ACT skills (particularly present-moment awareness and defusion)

Supportive staff team

Frequent contact via phone calls to supportive family members (surviving grandparents)

Engagement with volunteering opportunities – particularly gardening and outdoors ventures

Having regular and predictable one-to-one time with staff daily (pre-scheduled and always offered, even when little to talk about)

Identification of a place to call 'home' – stable accommodation

Support to address substance use (tailored to specific ID needs)

Exercise, fresh air, developing a meaningful sense of purpose and reason to get up in the morning

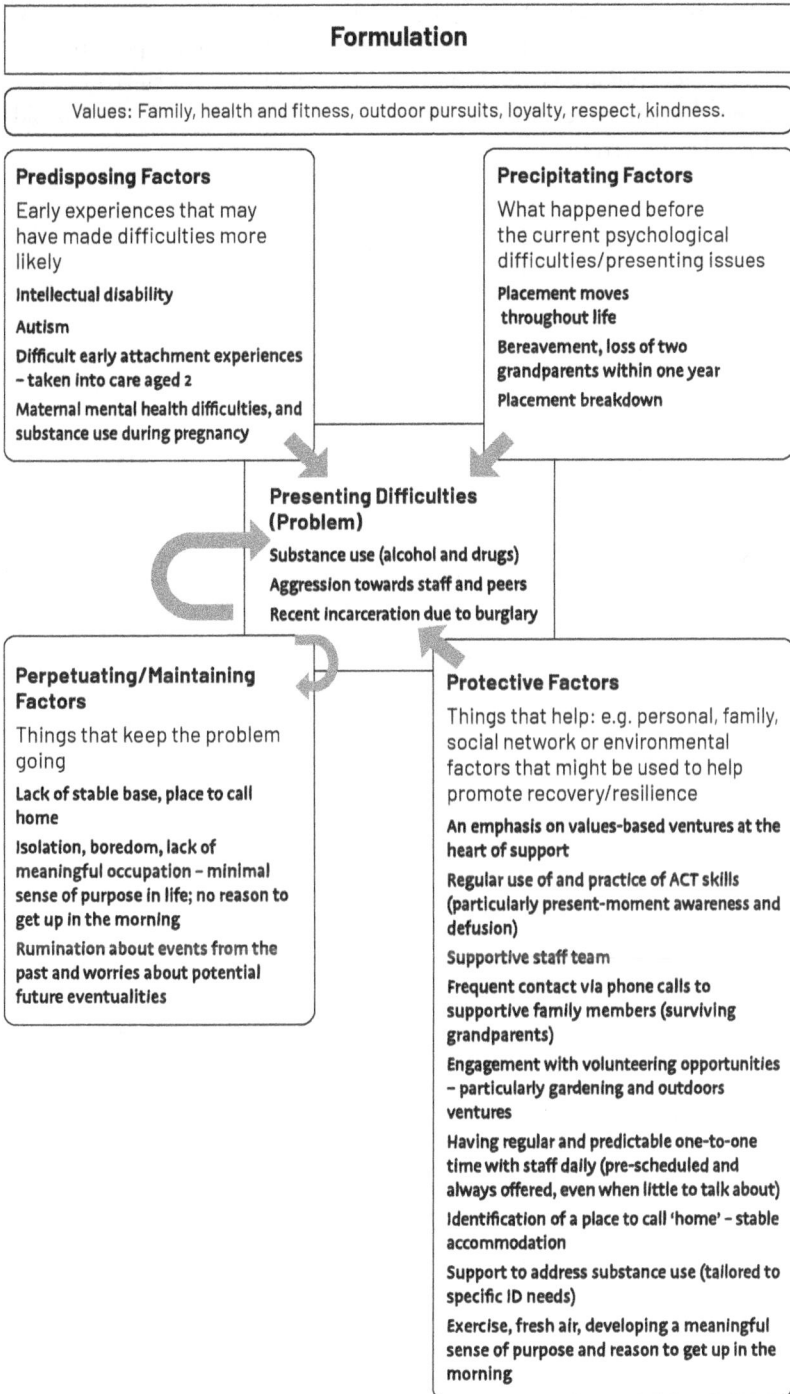

Figure 2.2b *An example of a collaboratively completed Five Ps formulation*

There are a number of other options for formulating within an ACT model: The Hexaflex can be used to consider the degree to which a person shows psychological flexibility in each of the six domains. Russ Harris has also developed a case conceptualization template which takes this into consideration (Harris, 2013).

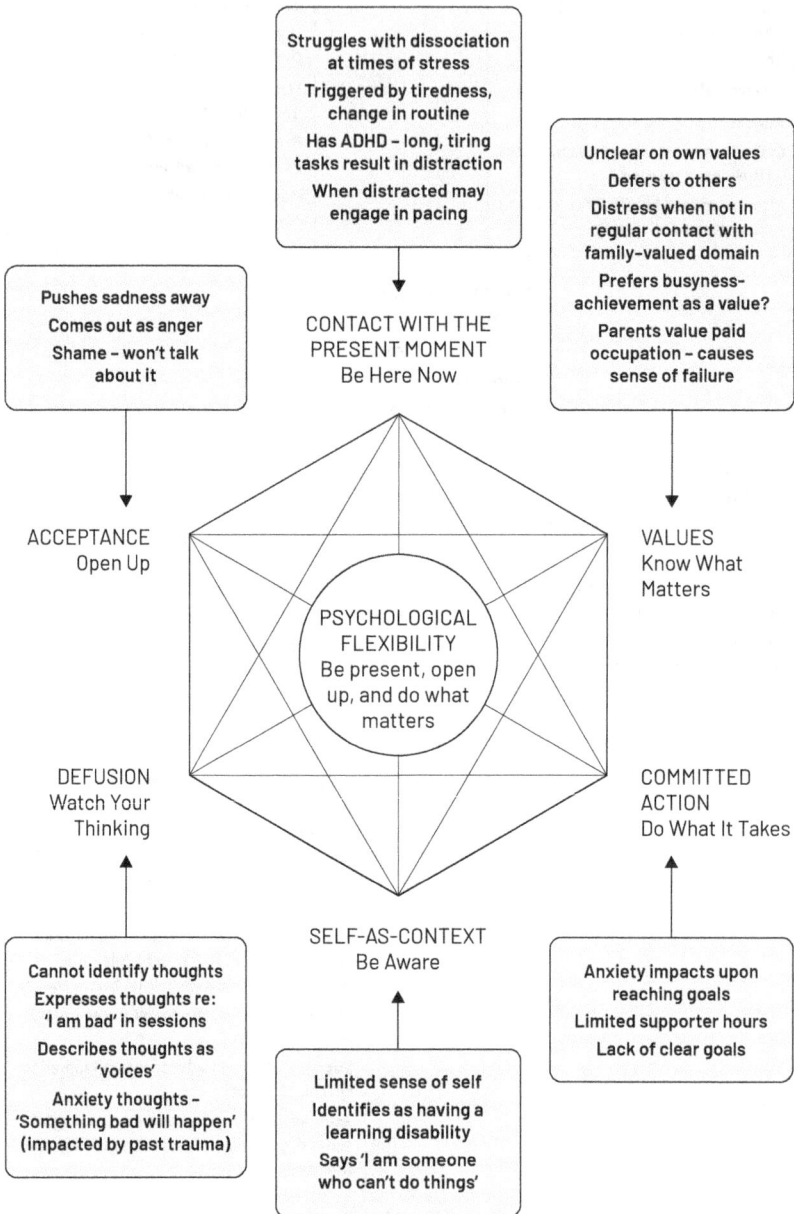

Struggles with dissociation at times of stress

Triggered by tiredness, change in routine

Has ADHD – long, tiring tasks result in distraction

When distracted may engage in pacing

Unclear on own values

Defers to others

Distress when not in regular contact with family-valued domain

Prefers busyness-achievement as a value?

Parents value paid occupation – causes sense of failure

Pushes sadness away

Comes out as anger

Shame – won't talk about it

CONTACT WITH THE PRESENT MOMENT
Be Here Now

ACCEPTANCE
Open Up

VALUES
Know What Matters

PSYCHOLOGICAL FLEXIBILITY
Be present, open up, and do what matters

DEFUSION
Watch Your Thinking

COMMITTED ACTION
Do What It Takes

Cannot identify thoughts

Expresses thoughts re: 'I am bad' in sessions

Describes thoughts as 'voices'

Anxiety thoughts – 'Something bad will happen' (impacted by past trauma)

SELF-AS-CONTEXT
Be Aware

Anxiety impacts upon reaching goals

Limited supporter hours

Lack of clear goals

Limited sense of self

Identifies as having a learning disability

Says 'I am someone who can't do things'

Figure 2.3 *Psychological flexibility Hexaflex*

Second, we have sometimes found it useful to use a CBT formulation model, for example the Beckian CBT formulation model (Beck, 1995) (Figure 2.4), – completing this and then considering areas of the Hexaflex that may be in operation within the various elements of the CBT formulation.

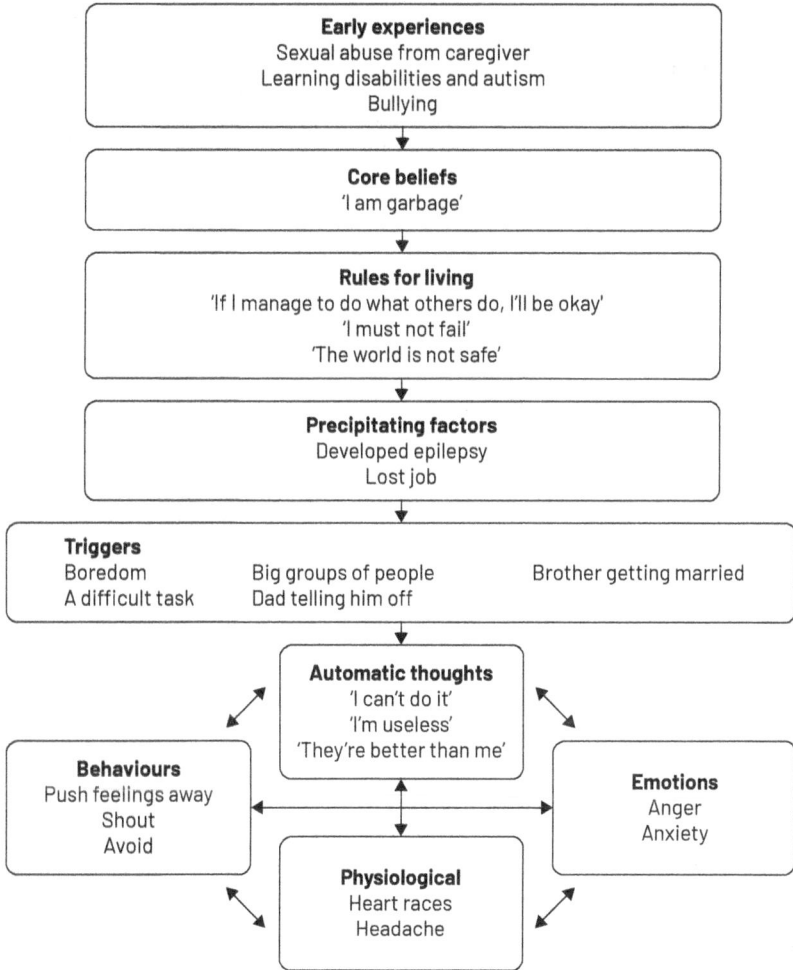

Early experiences
Sexual abuse from caregiver
Learning disabilities and autism
Bullying

Core beliefs
'I am garbage'

Rules for living
'If I manage to do what others do, I'll be okay'
'I must not fail'
'The world is not safe'

Precipitating factors
Developed epilepsy
Lost job

Triggers
Boredom   Big groups of people   Brother getting married
A difficult task   Dad telling him off

Automatic thoughts
'I can't do it'
'I'm useless'
'They're better than me'

Behaviours
Push feelings away
Shout
Avoid

Emotions
Anger
Anxiety

Physiological
Heart races
Headache

Figure 2.4 An example of Beckian CBT formulation

We also find Russ Harris's 'Choice Point' tool useful (Figure 2.5). The Choice Point is a visual tool used collaboratively to identify actions that are in accordance with one's values-based goals ('towards moves') and those that move the person away from these ('away moves'). It is also a tool to help identify thoughts and feelings that get in the way and strategies to overcome them. In Chapter 3 we discuss how to use this in an accessible way.

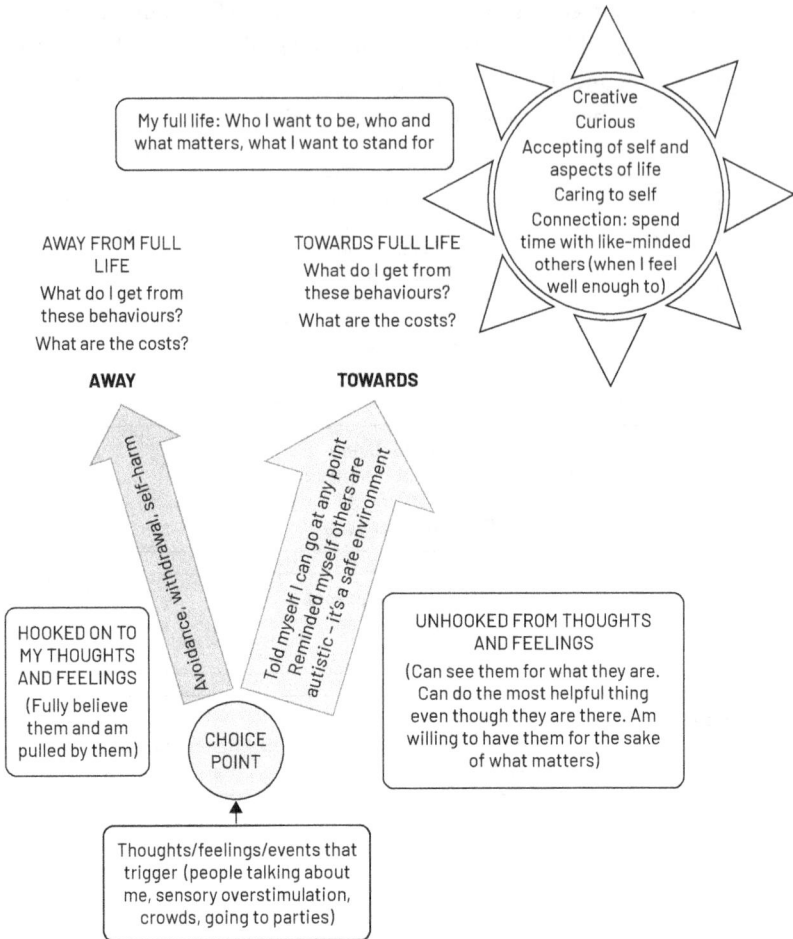

Figure 2.5 *The Choice Point*

Systemic formulation is extremely important when working therapeutically alongside people with intellectual disabilities. Systemic formulation considers the context, influence and dynamics present within the wider system. This should not be confused with (although the similar terms are confusing) systemic family therapy, which is something quite different altogether. Often, a person may have experienced a number of placement moves. There may be a lot of historical information that has either not yet been synthesized or has been lost during transitions. Therefore, systemic formulation plays a vital role in drawing together all aspects of an individual's case, of course with the individual remaining at the heart of this.

One model that encapsulates precisely this is the Complex Care and

Recovery Management (CCaRM) framework, developed by Spurrell, Potts and Shaw (2019, 2023). This can be very useful when working alongside multiple agencies and team members around a person with intellectual disabilities. The CCaRM offers a framework for working in meaningful partnership with people and their teams in relation to a broad range of care issues, with a particular focus on the things that truly matter to a person. The CCaRM therefore aligns particularly well with the ACT model, maintaining individual values at the heart of a systems-based formulation. A diagrammatic version of the CCaRM is shown in Figure 2.6.

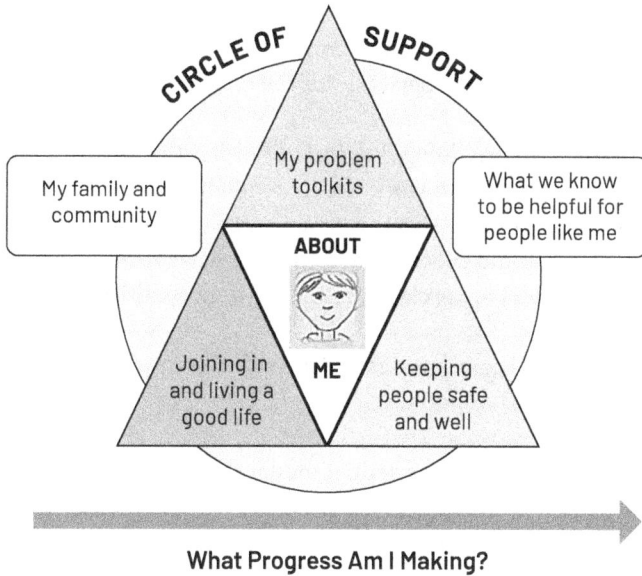

What Progress Am I Making?

Figure 2.6 The CCaRM framework (Spurrell, Potts & Shaw, 2023)

Finally, we also find using the Power Threat Meaning (PTM) framework (Johnstone & Boyle, 2018) useful. In brief the PTM framework offers an alternative to psychiatric diagnosis and, instead of working with diagnostic labels, asks:

1. What has happened to you? (How is power operating in your life?)
2. How did it affect you? (What kind of threats does this pose?)
3. What sense did you make of it? (What is the meaning of these situations and experiences to you?)
4. What did you have to do to survive?

Isn't ACT basically just CBT?

Cognitive behavioural therapy (CBT) is currently a ubiquitous therapy model in the UK. As ACT is a third-wave therapy, derived from second-wave therapies such as CBT, it can be useful to consider in which ways ACT and CBT differ from or are similar to each other.

Similarities to CBT include:

- Both focus on cognitive and behavioural aspects of situations, even if there are differences in the way these are approached.
- Both involve regular practice within real-life situations (homework).
- Therapy is structured, in the sense that there is an element of guidance from the practitioner (contrasting with the psychoanalytical tradition, where the person leads the content).

In ACT there is no pre-defined agenda or order: the key initial focus of any ACT intervention is to work closely to identify a person's values, the things that truly matter to them, with a view to then weaving in Hexaflex psychological skills and processes according to what arises in the moment, with the practitioner paying close attention to opportunities to practise each area of skill.

There are several core features that are either unique to or have a particular emphasis in ACT, especially:

- ACT is an active, experiential model that incorporates physicality and metaphor (e.g. the use of movement to explore experiences and stories to illustrate key points).

- ACT's overarching ethos is the promotion of psychological flexibility and acceptance in order to increase commitment to valued living (Hayes, Pistorello & Levin, 2012). Psychological flexibility is the ability to 'be present, open up and do what matters.' (Harris, 2019, p.12). This is a goal of ACT, whereas in CBT the goals relate to changing one's cognitions and/or behaviours in order to improve feelings.

- The focus of ACT is not on reduction in symptoms, but on creating a life full of meaning and value. This does *not* mean that reducing levels of significant distress is irrelevant, but that attention is moved to creating a life lived fully, even if that means some initial (or potentially ongoing) increase in anxiety.

- A central tenet of ACT is that the practitioner and person are 'in the same boat'. All humans suffer and struggle at times. It is not a sign of being in some way defective or needing to be fixed. The practitioner may use carefully considered self-disclosure and aims to model/use the key principles of ACT within therapy. There is also focus on the practitioner's own psychological flexibility and ability to model this in various areas of life.

- Attention is paid to the present moment; for example, the practitioner aims to identify cognitive and emotional changes within the therapy room and works with the person to aid them in noticing and sitting with such changes.

- ACT does not seek to identify irrational thinking and replace this with more balanced thinking, but explores 'workability' (simply, does it work to help the person live a values driven life?) with the person rather than whether something is objectively true or not. For example, does this behaviour, thought or action aid or hinder the person in their lives in moving towards valued aspects of life? Where thoughts are unworkable, the ACT approach is to consider ways to defuse from thoughts as opposed to altering them.

- ACT uses behavioural activation and exposure, both of which are used in CBT, but in ACT there is an explicit focus on values-based goals, and exposure in the service of values.

- In our experience, there is a motivational element to ACT; it is not only a talking therapy – the doing parts lead to change in unique ways. Whilst behavioural aspects of CBT also do so, we have found that experiential exercises within session have helped people to truly understand concepts and have galvanized them to make important changes in their lives.

Why use ACT for people with intellectual disabilities?

There is a strong rationale for using ACT with people with intellectual disabilities. Many people with intellectual disabilities have a complex support network, whether informal or formal, and goals may be set by supporters and support plans written by others. Behaviour support and risk plans may be well intentioned but focused on others' concerns. In this way, people with intellectual disabilities experience a lack of power in their lives, and it is easy for the person's values to become lost. The inherent focus upon values and workability in ACT helps to ensure that everyone (including the individual) knows and focuses on what matters most to the person, including the practitioner.

Requests for support can be made for a wide range of presenting difficulties. In our experience it is most commonly in areas such as anxiety, low mood, bereavement, behaviours that present challenges (e.g. aggression), self-esteem, obsessive/compulsive behaviours, feeling different to other people, or trauma. Since the Covid-19 pandemic, we have seen a significant rise in anxiety issues, such as repetitive and OCD-type behaviours. It is worth noting, however, that practitioners who work with people with intellectual disabilities do not solely work with mental health 'disorders'. Work may be needed in a variety of other areas, including sexuality and relationships, risk, emotional regulation, psychometric assessment, training of supporters, and much more. It is our experience that the ACT framework and philosophy can be useful in all of these areas, especially considering and incorporating the domain of Values, which underpins all of our work.

Fostering understanding

In the field of intellectual disabilities, there is a history of people's unusual or concerning actions being considered something that the person 'has' within them, or 'does' with intent. In fact, behaviours of all kinds are dependent on contextual or situational factors or serve some important function. Often, these actions are directed at an unmet need, even if those same actions do also cause difficulties for the person or those around them. The functional contextualist underpinnings of ACT help to shift the perspectives of supporters towards *understanding*. Understanding is a crucial facilitator of compassion. This shift to understanding naturally leads to supporters being more compassionate. They can then better support individuals to find more effective ways to achieve what they want in life.

As the following examples illustrate, the functional contextualism elements of an ACT approach are person-centred. This helps to take a person's life situation seriously, as well as considering their internal experiences, such as thoughts, emotions, goals and hopes, and still provides a scientific foundation to support change.

For example, understanding the function was crucial for Fatima:

CASE STUDY: Fatima

People thought Fatima was manipulative and reckless, because she would frequently offer her phone number to men with intellectual disabilities and agree to be their girlfriend, only to then ignore their calls and cause distress to many people. She would also enter risky situations with men and sometimes make subsequent false allegations. When understood within the framework of a history of being sexually exploited and abused by males, and of her behaviour having the function of an attempt to make herself safe (by pleasing men), supporters noted a drastic reduction in their feelings of frustration (which derived from a wish to keep her safe) and increase in compassion.

Similarly, but with a completely different function, understanding the underlying reason for distress was important for Chris:

CASE STUDY: Chris

Every evening during the winter, just after 4pm when the light faded outside, Chris's emotions would become heightened as indicated by raising his voice and shouting at staff and peers. Each time this occurred, staff would remove Chris from the communal lounge and take time to talk to him about the things on his mind. A thorough functional analysis indicated that Chris had a sensitivity to the bright lights that would be turned on every evening at dusk. By changing the lighting in the lounge area to a series of lamps, Chris was able to tolerate evening mealtimes and began to socialize in the evening once again without issue.

Focusing on values as a stable base within an unpredictable world

As we have said, people with intellectual disabilities are more likely to be exposed to traumatic life events than the general population (Hatton & Emerson, 2004), given the unique circumstances of their lives (Levitas & Gilson, 2001). Consequently, the identification of a consistent set of 'protective factors' (factors that help the person) for an individual may be difficult. Protective factors frequently draw on elements of life that lie outside of their control (such as engaging in activities or spending time with particular people). Protective factors may be transient and sometimes simply absent for people with intellectual disabilities for reasons that include loss, bereavement, financial problems and the political climate.

ACT encourages people to 'make room for life's difficulties' (Hayes et al., 1999, p.81) and move in the direction of their chosen values, even in the face of difficulty (Biglan, Hayes & Pistorello, 2008). ACT emphasizes individual ability to control some factors and not others; individuals are encouraged to exercise control in areas of life where control is likely to be effective (Hayes, 1994). The ability for people with intellectual disabilities and their support network to draw upon a readily available and easily accessible values system during times of adversity represents a key aspect of ACT. A focus upon supporting someone to develop a full life underpinned by a person's values and to maximize control in controllable areas will lead to improved social support, valued activities, skills development, and so on, which are well established protective factors that promote resilience and lead to improved mental health (Hayes, 2004).

Maintaining attention in sessions

Finally, the active element of ACT lends itself well to people with intellectual disabilities who may struggle to maintain conversation for long periods and with whom there can be a tendency to over-explain. It keeps the session interesting, dynamic and engaging for people highly likely to have attentional difficulties. ACT involves many different types of experiential exercises applied in a flexible way as the need arises. For example, rather than simply discussing mindfulness, mindfulness practices may be employed when a person appears to be less present; or where a person is fused with a thought, we may use Defusion exercises such as drawing or writing a thought (depending on the person's abilities) on a piece of paper.

The evidence base

There is an ever-growing evidence base for ACT interventions for the general population (Ost, 2014), especially for physical health conditions (Konstantinou et al., 2023). Indeed, the Association for Contextual Behavioral Science reported that there had been 1126 ACT-based randomized control trials as of June 2024. There is a developing evidence base for the use of ACT with people with intellectual disabilities (Byrne & O'Mahoney 2020; Gore & Hastings, 2016; Harper, Webb & Rayner, 2013; Leoni, Serafino, Cavagnola, 2015). However, as is the case for most psychological approaches in the intellectual disabilities field, there are not yet enough studies to draw confident conclusions, and the studies that do exist tend to be small-scale and lacking in robust research methodology.

It is important to distinguish between a lack of evidence and evidence of ineffectiveness. A lack of published studies does not mean ACT for people with intellectual disabilities is not effective (Osugo & Cooper, 2016). Byrne and O'Mahoney (2020) concluded that ACT interventions with people with intellectual disabilities were associated with reductions in psychological distress and improvements in adaptive skills. Findings suggest that further adaptations are required for ACT interventions for people with intellectual disabilities. Pankey and Hayes (2003, 2008) reported promising findings from a four-session, adapted individual ACT intervention for the treatment of psychosis in a female with intellectual disabilities, noting particular improvements in self-reported levels of distress. In a separate study, the effectiveness of a brief ACT group intervention for people with intellectual disabilities was demonstrated by Pankey and Hayes (2008), who reported increased psychological flexibility and time spent focused on important values and valued living.

A subsequent study by Brown and Hooper (2009) reported an adapted ACT intervention for the management of anxious, obsessive thoughts for a young person with moderate to severe intellectual disabilities. They noted that 'considerable adaptation' was required but found that after doing so the person's anxious thoughts had reduced in impact and they were able to return to college. Brown and Hooper (2009) also reported the challenges of facilitating the development of a sound understanding of the concept of 'values'.

Boulton, Williams and Jones (2018, 2020) reported on the use of photography to enhance accessibility of the concept of Values for six people with intellectual disabilities. This included development of a manualized therapeutic intervention delivered by three practitioners. Findings indicated that it is possible to isolate a single component of ACT and adapt it for use with people with intellectual disabilities. The study highlights the potential feasibility of a values-based approach for people with intellectual disabilities augmented through the use of photography to enhance accessibility. Boulton and colleagues noted some key findings, including:

- Participants with intellectual disabilities demonstrated an enhanced understanding of the concept of Values through the use of photography.
- Participants were able to report on their inner world by rating their levels of anxiety, experiential avoidance, mood and life satisfaction by successfully responding to text messages sent via an automated service using a camera-equipped mobile phone supplied by the research team.
- Participants embraced the use of photography. In-session exploration of captured photographs depicting valued aspects of life facilitated therapeutic focus and illustrated the concept of Values in a literal way.

A values-based intervention manual has since been designed specifically for people with intellectual disabilities. The *Catching What Matters*[1] intervention manual has been piloted with six participants with intellectual disabilities. The *Catching What Matters* intervention may be incorporated into sessions by practitioners to facilitate understanding of values-based concepts for people with intellectual disabilities and may be implemented with relative ease

---

[1]   A version of this manual is available by contacting the authors at pathnorthwest@ protonmail.com.

alongside (or by) supporters or staff teams. Positive feedback from trial practitioners has indicated that the intervention manual may form the basis of further development of future ACT-Intellectual Disability (ACT-ID) concepts.

Boddington and colleagues (2018) described the delivery of a nine-session ACT group intervention for adults with intellectual disabilities. The study included eight participants of which six completed the programme. Formal outcomes were not reported, but it was noted that group members provided positive feedback. Participants also reportedly struggled with the ACT concept of acceptance, preferring life difficulties to be eliminated. Simpler ideas, such as the 'quicksand' metaphor about struggling with emotions, worked better than somewhat more elaborate concepts, such as the (conceptually similar) 'unwelcome party guest' metaphor. Subsequently, Oliver et al. (2019) reported two case studies in which individuals with intellectual disability showed rapid improvement through the use of ACT.

Who can deliver ACT?

Therapies that involve expensive, time-consuming and tightly controlled accreditation pathways can be off the table for many professionals. Certainly, in the UK, especially in public services, funding for training is often scarce.

There is no accreditation process to become an ACT practitioner. In some ways we view this as hugely positive as it makes becoming skilled in ACT more accessible. That said, practitioners should not engage in using these therapies without the appropriate training and background. We recommend that practitioners using ACT principles should have at minimum attended a high-quality introductory course. They should also have access to supervision from a skilled ACT practitioner. Practitioners should exercise professional judgement around their own skill levels and continue to abide by the codes of conduct of their own core professional body.

Recommended reading

The fundamentals of ACT are detailed in several excellent books. For example: *ACT Made Simple* (2019), *The Happiness Trap* (2007) and *The Illustrated Happiness Trap* (2014), all by Russ Harris; *A Liberated Mind: The Essential Guide to ACT* (2019) by Steven Hayes; and *Acceptance and Commitment Therapy: The Process and Practice of Mindful Change* (2011) by Steven Hayes, Kirk Strosahl and Kelly Wilson (2011). Any of these would be a useful adjunct to this book.

There is also a range of excellent ACT-focused websites. For example, the Association of Contextual and Behavioral Science site has a wealth of useful resources for practitioners.[2] Again, accessing some good-quality training is highly recommended: ACT is an experiential therapy, and you really need to 'do it' to 'get it'.

There is only one ACT book for people with intellectual disabilities of which we are aware: *Living Your Best Life: Acceptance-Based Guided Self-Help for People with Intellectual Disabilities* (Williams & Jones, 2022), an ACT-based wellbeing workbook specifically for people with intellectual disabilities. This guided self-help style book covers the key elements of the ACT model. It includes sections on increasing wellbeing, and dealing with common challenges such as anxiety, low mood, anger difficulties, and bereavement.

SUMMARY

- Whilst there are similarities, ACT differs from CBT in some key ways: for example, in its approach to 'truth' versus 'workability'.

- ACT is experiential- and values-based, with a focus on developing a wholly lived life, rather than focusing primarily on symptom reduction.

- Aspects of ACT are very pertinent to therapeutic ventures alongside people with intellectual disabilities but also come with some challenges. Many of these can be overcome through a creative and flexibly tailored approach.

- ACT can be used individually or systemically with people with intellectual disabilities. The person-centred principles that are at the core of ACT are much needed for a group still marginalized and disempowered by society.

- More research is needed in the field of ACT for people with intellectual disabilities.

---

2   https://contextualscience.org

Chapter 3

PRINCIPLES OF ACCESSIBILITY

It is reasonably obvious we should use clear and simple language in therapeutic work with people with cognitive challenges. Nevertheless, it is common for practitioners to reflect on a piece of work and conclude that further adaptations would have been beneficial. On many occasions, despite apparently successful adaptations having been made, some concepts might not have been fully understood by the person. Many people with intellectual disabilities are adept at masking when they struggle with understanding, so it can easily be missed.

In this chapter, we provide an outline of key factors to bear in mind when considering therapeutic adaptations for people with intellectual disabilities. Some adaptations will be generally applicable, for example using simpler words, and giving more time to process information. However, the degree to which adaptations are made will need to be considered on an individual basis. Specific adaptations will be more suitable for some people than others, for example around the use of metaphors and visual aids. Individuals vary widely in their abilities according to, for example, their level of and type of intellectual disability, the presence of autism and any co-occurring difficulties (e.g. dyslexia, dyspraxia, physical ill health related to genetic conditions, to name a few). We also consider how to make adaptations specifically when using the ACT model, to take account of its unique elements.

It is important to consider the person's developmental level in different areas (Dagnan, Taylor & Burke, 2023). Some people may have undertaken a cognitive assessment or may have had some form of communication assessment from a speech therapist. This may help in considering the person's level of ability and profile of strengths and difficulties. Where these are absent and where practitioners are appropriately trained and confident in doing so, administering assessments of vocabulary can provide an estimate of a person's verbal ability that can help guide decisions about both appropriateness of therapy and ways in which to adapt it.

We find the Suitability for Engaging in Cognitive-Behavioural Therapy assessment tools useful (Dagnan, Chadwick & Proudlove, 2000). A similar 'pack' utilizing these and other tools was developed by Oathamshaw and Haddock (2006). These are visual tools that directly assess and train people in identifying emotions, thoughts and behaviours and the links between them. However, unless the person can identify only very few of these, the results should not necessarily preclude the person from engaging in therapy. Bruce and colleagues (2010) demonstrated that many people with intellectual disabilities can be taught the required skills to engage in CBT. An assessment may indicate that preparatory educative work is needed and can provide a useful roadmap for this.

An in-depth description of adaptations to CBT for people with intellectual disabilities is provided by Dagnan et al. (2023). Many of these adaptations can equally be applied to ACT. Dagnan et al. (2023) describe the need to consider:

- simplification
- consideration of language
- consideration of developmental level
- use of activities
- directive approaches
- flexibility
- context/involvement of supporters
- the therapeutic relationship and addressing disability.

We cannot assume that all ACT approaches will work with all people with intellectual disabilities. They need to be used tentatively and with clinical judgement based on an individual assessment. It is not always possible to predict which exercises will be effective. An element of adapting ACT will be the practitioner's ability to ascertain when practices or discussions are proving ineffective and to respond flexibly rather than slavishly persisting.

A directive approach

As Dagnan et al. (2023) describe, when engaging in therapy with people with intellectual disabilities there can be a greater need for the practitioner to offer structure and be appropriately directive. People may attend sessions without a clear idea of what to expect, what to talk about, or how they want the session to go. Some people may struggle to answer open questions and, in such cases, suggestions may need to be offered.

This can be aided by the collaborative development of an agenda, the practitioner having some plans for the session (approached flexibly), and having some structured exercises. That said, flexibility and responsiveness in the moment are equally important. It is certainly not sufficient to arrive at a session without any plans whatsoever. Whilst sessions may veer off course, a flexible agenda that has been developed together at the start of the session can be a handy reminder to check-in and make steps to get back on track, if appropriate.

We have developed agendas at the start of the session by asking the person we are working with to share the things they would like to focus on in the session. We write these on a flipchart. These could also be simply noted on a piece of paper on the table or stuck on the wall with sticky tape. Dependent on individual preference, this could even be noted on an iPad/tablet or drawn in picture format at the start of the session.

It can help you, and often also the individual you are working with, to set approximate times for each topic in the session. For example:

Example Session Agenda

- Catch-up and check in: how has the last week been? (Complete outcome rating scale.) – 5 minutes
- Agree agenda for today's session – 5 minutes
- Reflect on/work through difficulty from previous week – 15 minutes
- ACT skill development: practical exercise – 10 minutes
- Looking ahead to the next week: what do I have planned? (If very little, is there an opportunity to schedule in some low-key plans?) How can I use ACT skills to help me work through difficulties that may arise? – 10 minutes
- Bring session to a close, review key points from session and make plan for next session. (Complete session rating scale.) – 5 minutes

You can download outcome and session rating scales worksheets at https://digitalhub.jkp.com/redeem (or scan the QR code) using the voucher code UAHJYLC.

Cognitive and language considerations
Time to process information

Many people with an intellectual disability experience difficulties with speed of information processing. If the person has previously completed a cognitive assessment, it may be possible to access information about this and other cognitive abilities to inform your processing-related adaptations. The interpretation of cognitive assessments should only take place by appropriately qualified psychologists. However, in some cases a report will contain useful recommendations to consider at the outset of your work. Where such information is not available, be alert to the possibility of a slower speed of information processing. This could be shown as a delay in responding, or the person asking for repetition, which can also be a masking strategy.

Provide information at an appropriate pace. Avoid delivering more and more verbal information whilst a person is still processing the initial information. This can be difficult! Adapting one's speed may feel awkward or unfamiliar, compared with the usual pace of conversation. It may also not be immediately obvious to you that you are moving at too fast a pace. However, giving extra time is probably one of the most effective adaptations that a practitioner can make. It can also help to check out the person's understanding at regular intervals, particularly when conveying complex information. This offers an opportunity for the individual to repeat back their interpretation of the information that you have so far shared.

It is good practice to initially avoid 'jumping in' during therapy. Allow the person to form their own conclusions and make sense of their situations, without being disempowered by someone offering their 'expert' advice. But stepping in and offering suggestions may be needed where people are struggling to do this independently.

Avoiding overload

Many people with intellectual disabilities experience difficulties with working memory. Working memory is the ability to hold various pieces of information in mind, whilst at the same time using that information to compute a response (Baddeley, 1986).

Presenting information in 'bite-size chunks' can be extremely helpful. This involves describing one principle or request at a time. Cut out unnecessary words and information in each sentence. For example, when we deliver ACT in a group setting, only one new concept is introduced in each session (e.g. *watching your thoughts* or *doing what matters*). We would recommend the same during individual work.

This is supported by Dagnan et al. (2023), who emphasize the importance of repetition and being alert to fatigue. Indicators of fatigue may be subtle, and often unique to each individual. Tune in to these signs through discussion at the start of sessions with the individual or alongside supporters. In our experience, signs of fatigue in sessions include the obvious – yawning, stretching and eye rubbing – to more subtle indicators such as looking out of the window, checking the time, frequent changes of subject, general agitation or apparent disengagement.

CASE STUDY: Stan

Within a clinical setting, one of us has experienced Stan almost dozing off during discussion of difficult concepts. If something like this happens, think about terminating the session. Where relevant, communicate the issue to supporters for monitoring. In this case, the fatigue was indicative of issues related to prescribed medication side-effects.

The primary issue of the medication could be addressed alongside tailoring session times to best suit Stan. For example, we could avoid sessions after daytime activities such as college. Sessions could be scheduled into points in the week where less demand was placed on Stan, such as the morning of their day off from routine activities.

Visual support

Dagnan et al. (2023) summarize a range of recommendations about communication style, including keeping sentences short and avoiding words of greater than three syllables. Lots of people with intellectual disabilities also find visual aids useful in understanding different concepts and retaining information for future use. Visuals can be especially important when a person has no, or limited, reading ability, or problems with working memory. However, the utility of visual aids is not limited to those situations. Many autistic people are 'visual thinkers', and they and others will benefit from visual material, regardless of their intellectual abilities.

Visual aids can come in the form of 'off-the-shelf' pictures to demonstrate particular ACT principles but can also involve bespoke in-session drawing of ACT-related concepts relevant to the discussions. As described previously, photographs taken by individuals themselves and brought along to sessions have been demonstrated to be a particularly useful way to establish a person's values, as well as a way to monitor the extent to which an individual is making choices to move towards value aspects of life (Boulton, Williams & Jones, 2018).

It can often be useful to ensure any agenda made at the start of the session is visible for the duration of the session. If agreed at the outset, it can also be helpful to 'tick off' each section once complete. This provides a visual overview of progress made during session and works towards keeping the session on track. This approach may not be for everyone, so do check within early sessions as to whether this may be a suitable approach. It may also be the case that agenda items to be 'rolled over' may be less relevant for the individual in the next session. If so, it can be helpful to reflect on ways that this issue may have been resolved. Often, praise may be provided for the effective implementation of problem-solving or newly learned ACT skills!

Some examples of visual aids within therapy contexts:

- Flipcharts, thought/speech bubbles to represent possible interpretations of events/noticing thoughts; introduction of physical objects to make abstract concepts concrete.

- Painting/modelling with clay, cutting out pictures from magazines/ participant-produced photographs, making a collage to represent aspects of the ACT psychological flexibility model. Aspects of a collage may be collected collaboratively during the session. This can be done through shared use of a computer and searching for images that are relatable for the individual, or perhaps from magazines or catalogues.

- A 'session tracker' such as a pie chart divided into the total number of planned sessions, shaded by the person at the end of each session to represent completion.

- Using smartphone features, such as apps, notes sections, calendars and voice recorders. Using 'notes' on a smartphone to depict a collaboratively agreed agenda, the 'tick' emoji can also be used together once a section has been completed. This is a positive way of highlighting progress as well as being clear about which aspects of the planned agenda may be rolled over to the next session if further discussion is required.

Not everyone is a visual thinker or learner. Some people may feel offended or patronized by pictorial aids. Check what the person themselves finds helpful. Many people may not be clear on their own learning style but will be able to feed back on whether they like particular visual aids. During the early stages of the therapy, have conversations to elicit feedback about visual materials.

Retention

As with any therapy, individuals may struggle to retain information pertaining to the topics covered within sessions. However, by using the ACT model, this issue is somewhat ameliorated since ACT is more about *doing* than talking and naturally incorporates lots of experiential and/or visual exercises that will aid memory.

Some suggestions to aid memory:

- audio or mobile phone recordings as an alternative to literacy based therapeutic activities
- home-tasks, personal diary records and easy-read handouts to facilitate between-session generalization (i.e. the ability to apply learning from sessions to real-life scenarios when required)
- use of repetition
- use of experiential exercises, supplemented by repetition about the point of the exercise
- videos (e.g. therapists may direct individuals to helpful videos on YouTube or ones the therapist has developed themselves to explain a concept); individuals may watch these between sessions, alongside supporters, where appropriate; this enhances generalisability of concepts
- help from supporters with between-session practice.

Recognizing thoughts

It may be difficult for many people to recognize that their thoughts are indeed thoughts, as opposed to an unquestioned narration of reality.

A common early position within therapy is often *If I think something, it must be true.* It can take some time to move towards a position of *Just because I think something, it doesn't make it true.* This is a particular difficulty for some people who struggle to think at a 'metacognitive' level. (Metacognition is an awareness of one's own thought processes and insight into the patterns around them.)

CASE STUDY: Tim

Over time, Tim recognized that his anxiety about having worrying thoughts had prevented him from doing many of the things that he had previously loved, such as playing five-a-side football with his friends. Through this recognition, Tim was able to rationalize that worrying thoughts may come and go; he can *choose* whether to let these prevent him from doing the things that are important to him, or to feel the fear and move towards values aspects of life anyway. This enabled him to return to this activity and manage when such thoughts occurred.

Many people with intellectual disabilities verbalize their thoughts in the form of self-talk. So, we might sometimes describe thoughts as 'words that pop into your head' or 'words that you say to yourself'. There may need to be considerable time spent training people to catch their thoughts as they arise. This can be done as an explicit exercise but should also be done as the thoughts arise and are verbalized by the person in session (i.e. 'catching' and naming thoughts that the person says out loud in the session). This can be much more effective than expecting the person to recall their thoughts from several days ago.

Further guidance around working with thoughts can be found in the Defusion section in Chapter 6.

Understanding emotions

People with intellectual disabilities often experience difficulties not only with emotion regulation but also understanding and recognizing emotions. Without preliminary work in this area, there is a risk that engagement with sessions may be superficial, posing a risk that one may 'lose' the person from the outset. To experience and accept a difficult feeling, a person must first identify it. Do not assume that the person can identify a range of emotions or that they can link emotions to thoughts and behaviours.

The Contact with the Present Moment and Acceptance domains of the ACT models contain practices that may help people enhance their emotional literacy. In working with people with intellectual disabilities it is usually necessary to include more work around emotion recognition than is described in typical ACT approaches and publications. In this book, these elements are included as part of a 'toolkit' of skills. We have found body maps useful: activated areas of the body associated with emotions are shown (Nummenmaa et al., 2014). The person can draw on a body map based on their own experiences, if they are willing. A thorough assessment and education (if needed) will enable you to specifically tailor your intervention to an individual's level of ability and understanding and prepare someone for engaging in ACT.

Insight

In basic terms, insight can be thought of as recognizing one's difficulties (and strengths) and understanding the links between attempts to cope with difficulties and the results of these coping attempts. For example, a person struggling with traumatic memories is able to understand that they are using alcohol as a means of coping with their intrusive memories and feelings of shame.

A person's insight into the workability of their behaviours can sometimes be affected by memory or their ability to reflect and work at a metacognitive level. Additional work and support around insight may therefore be required to tease out what is or is not workable for the person. However, it is important to establish whether there is simply a difference in values between the person and the practitioner, as opposed to a case of limited insight.

For example, an overweight person may say that comfort eating is not a problem for them. This may indeed be true. Physical health may not be an important value for the person, as they may be within a context where eating unhealthy food is normal. But it could also be that the person has not yet developed insight into the links between their behaviours and the long-term consequences on valued living. Where this is the case, work may be needed on encouraging the person to be more aware of the links. This could involve the use of diaries, or additional information highlighting the links between actions and particular outcomes. Once you are satisfied that someone has sufficient insight (or capacity) into their behaviours, you can feel more confident that they can make informed choices about their actions. Where a person may be then making what appear to be unwise decisions, for example in relation to their lifestyle, as a practitioner you will need to be accepting of choices that you feel are harmful in some way.

In supporting insight, it can be helpful to deliver psychoeducation about our evolved human instincts. This helps to normalize and reduce feelings of shame: for example, describing in appropriately accessible terms how people are designed to choose short-term over longer-term gains because day-to-day decisions were life and death for our ancient ancestors. Similarly, because it was important to ensure there was enough daily food (energy) and water available for everyone, we have evolved to find and eat high energy foods. In order to help with the common difficulty of obesity (in wealthier parts of the world), we need to help people to strengthen links between longer-term adaptive behaviours and the shorter-term, small, moment-to-moment actions that will form the path to those longer-term goals.

Some people struggle to consider the longer-term consequences. Exercises that break down longer-term goals into smaller steps can be helpful. Conceptualize goals as short-term, medium-term and long-term, homing in on the smaller stepping stones along the way towards achieving these. For example, a long-term goal may be to *get a job in a shop*, but a short-term goal towards this may be *work on getting up in the morning*, whereas a medium-term goal might be *practise job interviews*. As another example, a person who values connection with others could begin to contact old friends or say hello to people in their local area, with the practitioner normalizing and acknowledging the longer-term time and effort involved in the goal of developing good connections.

Suggestibility

Suggestibility is defined as 'an inclination to readily and uncritically adopt the ideas, beliefs, attitudes or actions of others' (American Psychological Association, 2018). Humans can tend towards suggestibility, probably because we have evolved to function as part of small tribes. Getting along with those tribes was key to survival, since being outcast from the tribe would have meant certain death. So, being suggestible at certain times may have had evolutionary advantages (a 'workable' strategy).

However, in modern times, this is less useful to us. Suggestibility can be problematic. It can lead to people being exploited or denying their own needs and wishes for the sake of others and to their own detriment. People with intellectual disabilities often find themselves in a position of being surrounded by people who are more verbally and cognitively able, so it is no surprise that suggestibility can be common (Gudjonsson & Henry, 2003). It can be an effective way to mask difficulties with understanding, reduce feelings of awkwardness or shame and maximize the chance of acceptance, despite carrying significant disadvantages.

Consider and monitor for suggestibility, since this can have an impact on the long-term success and meaningful impact of interventions. We have had experience of suggestibility leading to some exercises being ineffective in their aim. One ACT exercise designed to illustrate that thoughts do not have to equate to action involves demonstrating to the person how the therapist 'installing' a thought in their mind (e.g. asking them to raise their arm up) does not have to equate to said action. However, we have experienced that some people *will* lift their arm, so we use other ways to demonstrate this point.

Use of metaphor

The use of verbal and visual metaphor also requires careful consideration with people with intellectual disabilities (Shnitzer-Meirovich, Lifshitz-Vahab & Mashal, 2017, cited in Dagnan et al., 2023). With some individuals, particularly some autistic people, it may be most helpful to avoid metaphors altogether. Their level of concrete thinking may mean they are unable to hold in mind the metaphor and compare with another scenario. Whilst ACT typically relies on metaphorical language in an effort to expand or extend behavioural repertoires, people with intellectual disabilities 'can often present with very limited abilities to reason beyond a very concrete and linear understanding of thoughts and events' (Pankey & Hayes, 2008, p.29). Fortunately, it is still possible to utilize ACT without metaphor.

However, some people can make very good use of tailored metaphors. There are many ACT metaphors provided on video-sharing platforms or within key ACT textbooks. For example, 'passengers on the bus' is a metaphor for which there is a very useful animation on YouTube. The metaphor is one of a bus driver (representing the person), who is driving down the 'same old road' (non-values-based and less fulfilling life), and when attempting to drive down a new, unfamiliar, but exciting and fun road (representing a values-based life), his/her passengers (representing thoughts/feelings) become angry, pressuring them to stop. For people who understand this metaphor, the idea of naming the passengers (e.g. 'my angry passenger is telling me to hit out') can be useful.

'Demons on the boat' is another useful metaphor. It depicts travelling on a boat, sailing towards a desired location (values-based goals) whilst being chased by demons (difficult thoughts, feelings and so on). The demons cannot harm but can be intimidating while the person sails towards their destination.

Visual aids can be more effective than verbally describing concepts or metaphors. They can reduce the requirement to hold multiple pieces of information in one's head (working memory) and can be an engaging way in which to illustrate concepts. In some cases, it can be useful to pause video sections and explain the comparisons at different points. Ensure that you discuss explicitly how the metaphor may relate to the person. Don't expect the person to automatically make those links and be able to apply the principles in their own life.

The complexity of metaphors should also be matched to the ability of the person to think abstractly, although that is no guarantee that the specific metaphor will be understood. It is also helpful to use metaphors that are meaningful in the person's world. These should be co-constructed as much as possible, developed together in session and based on personal interests. For example, use characters from favourite television shows, concepts linked to a person's special interests, such as vehicles or fairground rides, and so on. This can be especially useful for people who have hyper-focused interests.

The use of special interests is described in further detail when we consider the case of Catherine in Chapter 4. Catherine loved musical theatre. The analogy of the Yellow Brick Road from the film *The Wizard of Oz* really helped her to conceptualize moving towards her values using the Choice Point, despite inevitable twists and turns on the path of life.

We have used metaphors to good effect on many occasions, and in others have been less successful – it really does vary with individuals! We have used a 'climbing the mountain' metaphor to illustrate the importance of Committed Action ('You don't know what's at the top of the mountain until you get there'), to which a person's response was 'But I don't climb mountains' (literal interpretation).

Some people understand and can apply the 'passengers on the bus' metaphor, whereas others continue to only recall the bus or other concrete details of the metaphor. One individual stated that they learnt from the metaphor to 'not distract the driver', showing a misunderstanding of the concept, perhaps due to level of complexity. Others have enjoyed the metaphor and spontaneously linked it to areas of their life. There is no blanket rule as to who can understand metaphors. You may need to test this out to know for sure.

If videos are not used, we recommend other types of visuals. This could be a picture, or a drawing created within the session. You could even use a miniature bus and figures to illustrate the 'passengers on the bus' metaphor. Pictures and drawings are helpful because people can take these away with them (or a photo of them taken on their mobile phone) to help with memory retention and prompting.

Checking understanding

The need for regularly checking the person's understanding during sessions cannot be overstated. Many people with intellectual disabilities have learnt to acquiesce and mask their lack of understanding, due to feelings of shame and inadequacy.

The emphasis in ACT on us 'all being in the same boat' fits well with the need to help people to move out of shame to a place of self-acceptance. Normalize how confusing and difficult therapy can be. Ask 'Have I explained this properly?' rather than 'Did you understand that?' Ask the person what they took from the conversation, without appearing to be testing the person.

The nuances of ACT can be difficult to grasp, and it is easy for the person to misunderstand. We have experienced people who have interpreted acceptance to mean 'I should just put up with it'. Where such a message has been heard, it has not been delivered/interpreted correctly. Clarification, repetition, visual aids and, as ever, having a trusting and safe therapeutic relationship are needed, so that the person feels free to say if they have not understood or are confused.

Neurodiversity

The term *neurodiversity* is used to encapsulate a wide range of neurodivergent conditions, including autism, ADHD, dyspraxia, dyslexia and dyscalculia. Around one in three people with intellectual disabilities also have an autism spectrum condition (Rydzewska et al., 2018) and around three-quarters of people with an autism spectrum disorder have co-morbid ADD/ADHD (Rong et al., 2021). Therefore, it is important to consider salient issues and specific adaptations for this subgroup of individuals with intellectual disabilities. In the UK, the Equality Act 2010 makes it a statutory requirement for services to make reasonable adjustments for someone with autism, as well as for people with disabilities more generally, including intellectual disabilities.

A range of challenges are experienced by people who are neurodivergent. For example, processing difficulties can lead to information overload. Sensory difficulties can lead to feeling overwhelmed. High levels of anxiety and depression are experienced by many autistic people (Hollocks et al., 2019). 'Masking' is a commonly used strategy for coping with aversive situations. Some autistic people suppress their own thoughts and feelings about what matters to them in order to attempt to fit in (assimilation), whereas others may actively compensate (e.g. by copying). We should explore any additional neurodivergence that someone with an intellectual disability may have and consider specific adaptations that may be required during therapy. Whilst there are many types of neurodivergence, we focus particularly on autism and ADHD, which are the most common forms we encounter.

We advocate adopting a neuro-affirmative approach. As with neurotypical people, all autistic people are unique and will have different strengths and needs. Autistic people will have varying degrees of differences in how they manage change, understand the minds of others and communicate.

This variation increases when someone has an additional intellectual disability, as the traits linked to autism interact with the person's areas of cognitive strengths and difficulties. It is important to consider that autism represents a different way of being rather than something that is 'less than'. With it comes many strengths that someone who is neurotypical is less likely to have. For example, some people have an ability to focus on detail and favoured tasks, an affinity for structures and order, and different world perspectives that can create more original and innovative thinking. It is beyond the scope of this book to give a comprehensive guide, but there are already some excellent resources that can be accessed via the Autistic Research Collective or (in the UK) the National Autistic Society.

Whilst noting the need for individual formulation, there are some key principles to bear in mind in working with autistic people:

- *Allow for sensory and environmental issues, such as noise, lights or a cluttered environment*: Check these elements out with the person. Graded exposure is likely not to be helpful for sensory issues, so sensory issues need to be carefully picked apart from learned anxieties.

- *Pay attention to waiting rooms*: Is there clear signage and provision of sensory items in the waiting room (e.g. fidget spinners, glitter balls, soft blankets)? Ensure the waiting period is kept to a minimum; be clear on what to do on arrival; have a quieter area available if required.

- *Recognize the 'double empathy problem'* (Milton, 2012): Rather than locating a problem within the person, recognize that if the practitioner is neurotypical, communication with a neurodivergent person may have inherent challenges to overcome. Both parties may have difficulty understanding each other's thoughts, feelings, behaviours and differences. Where possible/appropriate try to discuss this as an issue and discuss communication styles.
    - As a practitioner, do not make assumptions based on non-verbal or verbal communication. If someone is not smiling, this does not necessarily mean they are not experiencing happiness or pleasure at that moment. Equally, if an individual appears to show a willingness to attend therapy and seemingly engages with the process from week to week yet avoids eye contact for the duration of all sessions, don't assume that this indicates an avoidance of fully engaging in the therapeutic process. This may be an aspect of their autism that influences their presentation.
    - Together, be curious, open and transparent from the outset. Encourage an open dialogue on both sides to begin to address the potential double empathy problem.

- *Alleviate anxiety about engaging in therapy*: Therapy involves talking intensely to a stranger for up to an hour. As a result, some people will engage in masking in the therapy room, to fit in, do the 'right thing' and please the practitioner. Unless addressed, this can be a barrier to therapy. Helping the person to feel safe, understood and validated, and explicitly stating permission to engage in behaviours that make the person feel comfortable in the room can help: for example, autistic behaviours such as stimming (this is a term often used to describe a repetitive action/movement that helps someone self regulate).

- *Be clear and transparent*: It is important that the practitioner does not assume the person knows what you are thinking or feeling based on your body language. Be literal/explicit about how therapy works, and clear in any communication, both written and verbal.

- *Provide written summaries*: These can be very helpful following a session. Some people will struggle to retain the discussions or any key points.

- *Offer soothing items*: Items such as fidget spinners may help some people to manage their anxiety. Some people prefer to bring their own items (e.g. a special object to offer comfort during the session).

- *Bring a person's particular interests into therapy*: Using metaphors, examples or visual tools related to a person's interests can help with focus and engagement and make the activity more meaningful.

- *Pay particular attention to motivation factors*: It is important that people are able to see links, for example, between behaviours and mood; without this, people may lack motivation to engage.

- *Recognize and adapt to alexithymia*: Up to 50 percent of people with autism have some degree of alexithymia, the inability to notice and name emotions (Kinnaird, Stewart & Tchanturia, 2019). Asking someone how they feel may be difficult and therefore anxiety-provoking. If this is the case, try asking the person 'What can you notice in your body?' or show body maps/feelings wheels as guides. You may wish to enlist the support of a trained speech and language therapist, when this option is available.

- *Make things predictable*: Predictability is important for the vast majority of autistic people. Create routine and give prior information. This may include sending out detailed information about the appointment beforehand, keeping appointments to a set time, informing people about the structure of sessions as early as possible, and ensuring people are warned as far in advance as possible about any changes.

- *Provide information that is concrete, clear and unambiguous*: You may need to slow down the pace of sessions and allow extra time and longer sessions to take processing difficulties into account.

Whilst there are certainly some challenges in using ACT to support autistic people, in many other ways ACT lends itself very well. It is often guided, structured (albeit with flexibility built in) and focused on exercises and activities. This reduces the demands on intense communication and prolonged eye contact. As a core trait of autism is rigidity of thinking; learning how to become more psychologically flexible through ACT can be very helpful.

Hyperactivity and inattention

Sometimes, difficulties such as hyperactivity and inattention, common in, but not exclusive to, ADHD are given less consideration than other aspects of neurodiversity. They also sometimes remain undiagnosed. One adaptation is to have shorter sessions, or within a typical one-hour therapy session, to include plenty of opportunities for breaks

It may also be helpful to break up sessions with different types of activities, such as exercises that involve movement and a focus on emotion regulation, such as mindful breathing and grounding techniques. Some individuals may also enjoy working together with felt-tip pens and paper to draw out concepts whilst discussing during the session. This is a strategy that we have used previously: no judgements are made regarding drawing abilities – everything is welcomed! Collaboratively developing a session structure and plan at the start, with regular check-ins, supports focus and assists ability to conceptualize progress as the session continues.

A recent development among the ADHD community is the practice of body doubling. A person with ADHD completes a task (often a potentially frustrating task, such as dealing with paperwork, or doing household chores) alongside another person. This other person acts as the 'body double' for the person with ADHD. The role of the body double is to support orientation to the present moment and focus on the task in hand, acting as an anchor point with the aim of reducing the risk of distraction. Anecdotal evidence appears to indicate that the mere presence of a body double can help to soothe an anxious mind. A calm presence of another person may also support role-modelling of attentive and focused work.

Whilst there is currently limited formal evidence regarding the effectiveness of body doubling, this is a strategy that may be adopted within the therapeutic space, as well as between sessions, to support generalization of ACT strategies and principles. A person may practise strategies alongside a supporter. Creative methods such as the therapist recording snippets of advice or activities on a person's mobile phone may be used to support this both in and out of sessions.

Important factors to consider

Who wants change?

In working therapeutically with people with intellectual disabilities, consider *who* it is that wants the therapy. It is common for supporters or professionals to identify a problem area for the person, while the person themselves may feel ambivalent, or lack understanding around why they have been brought to therapy. They may not even have been asked their feelings about therapy at all.

Sometimes, the person is brought to a session by a supporter with an expectation or hope that the practitioner will 'fix' the person. Providing consent has been given, this expectation may be less of an issue where a difficulty is in fact easily 'treated', but it can be unrealistic and constitute (albeit usually well-intentioned) wishful thinking.

Part of the assessment should be to consider *who* is wanting change, *where* power is operating, and *how* motivated the person with intellectual disabilities is to attend therapy. The practitioner should seek to avoid colluding with any power imbalances. They should aim to understand the person's degree of motivation, understanding and willingness to be in the therapy room.

Method of adaptation

Rather than starting from the perspective of a standard ACT intervention and working back to make this more accessible, try to distil the core features of a particular concept. Then consider concept, and then consider what is needed to help a particular individual engage with a concept or technique.

For example, when considering Self-as-Context, there are several metaphors that have been suggested in non-adapted ACT (e.g. 'You are the sky, your thoughts [or insert another process] are the weather' or 'Your roles/life/ behaviour are the chess pieces, you are the chess board'). We tend to avoid these as they are too abstract for most people we have worked with. We certainly would not refer to chess, which would be outside of most people's experience.

Instead, we have considered:

* what areas in relation to sense of self are most pertinent to people with intellectual disabilities (e.g. self-esteem and an enhanced appreciation of the various roles and aspects of their self they take on)[1]
* how we support people to work on these areas.

---

1   More detail on this is given in the 'Self-as-Context' section in Chapter 6, as this is provided here more as an example of the process of adaptation rather than about the content.

Working on sense of self and enhancing people's appreciation of the various roles they can take has tended to be most pertinent and helpful. Some people with learning disabilities can have fixed negative views of themselves as not being capable. In such cases, consider roles they have taken where they have shown capability.

Similarly, it can be helpful to support a person to consider times they have demonstrated certain valued characteristics, such as being kind, making someone laugh or being a good friend, alongside features of each that contributed to the characteristics. For example: 'I was kind when I held the door open for a person in the shop;' 'I was a good friend when I asked how my friend's day at work had been.'

Body-/action-focused approaches

As we have said, one of the reasons that ACT lends itself well as a therapy model for people with intellectual disabilities is the emphasis on experience rather than talking. This enables people to discover important insights for themselves in a felt sense, not only in a cognitive sense. Dagnan and colleagues (2023) also described the utility of activities, as opposed to verbal interchanges, to explore ideas.

Check that the person knows about, and consents to, engaging in practical exercises from the start. Provide some information about any experiential exercises before you do them, without going into too much depth, since ACT is more about doing than talking. Some people can have high anxiety about unexpected events, so understanding what will happen next and being invited to take part, rather than feeling coerced, may help significantly. This is also consistent with a trauma-informed approach, which emphasizes fostering a sense of safety.

Some people will benefit from integrating interest in art, drama or music into the exercises. It can be helpful to use role-play to explore emotions and outcomes and to practise using skills in a range of potential scenarios. Perhaps an individual may wish to role-play different characters from a favourite show or topic of special interest. The presence of supporters during such ventures may aid generalization to real-life situations beyond the therapy space, because supporters will be educated about the skills and strategies being practised and will be more able to prompt the person to recall and use them when needed. 'Self-modelling' can be useful as well, whereby the person may develop and view a film of themselves engaging in desired behaviours and valued activities (Murphy & Davis, 2005). There are also a variety of practical mindfulness exercises to enhance understanding and appreciation of concepts such as mindful walking, blowing bubbles, soles-of-the-feet meditation

(Singh et al., 2011), and mindful eating (Chapter 6). Action-oriented experiential approaches are discussed in more detail later.

Involving supporters

It is common to involve family or paid supporters at some point in adapted ACT therapy, since they can be of enormous value in aiding the application and generalization of the session content. How much this is required will depend both on the wishes of the person with intellectual disabilities and the therapeutic need. This is an important decision to be made in the assessment phase. Some people will want a supporter to be present for the entire session due to their level of anxiety or for other reasons. This may change as the therapeutic relationship develops.

It can sometimes be helpful to invite the supporter into a session at the end, to summarize and clarify any role they may take. Consider asking the person themselves to summarize key points from the session to the supporter. This provides a natural way to establish how much the person has understood and taken from the session. It is more enabling too, unless of course they do not feel confident enough and would prefer you to do it.

This can also offer an opportunity for the person to share any aspects that may have been less well understood, and to work through this with the assistance of their supporter. This end-of-session summary can be a good time to discuss any between-session (home) practice. It is generally better to avoid the term 'homework', as this has negative connotations for many people. Involvement from supporters can also provide useful information about any systemic factors that may need to be considered separately: for example, insight into the relationship between the person and their supporter(s). This will be elaborated on in Chapter 10.

As Dagnan and colleagues (2023) state, there are challenges to involving supporters that the practitioner may need to attend to. These include keeping the person central to the session rather than the supporters' concerns becoming central, ensuring the supporters are clear on their role, and ensuring the person feels sufficiently empowered to participate fully.

Tolerating doing something new

As practitioners, we are not immune to the need to protect people with intellectual disabilities from distress. However, we must be willing to manage our own anxiety and discomfort in supporting the person to do unfamiliar experiential exercises in sessions, where both parties may feel somewhat out of their comfort zone. Otherwise, we fail to model the very principles of ACT we hope to convey. All kinds of practitioner fears may arise regarding the person's experience, yet taking a leap of faith is where change can sometimes occur the most. In taking risks that may facilitate change, we model the ability to make ourselves vulnerable and remind the person that we, too, are flawed humans who make mistakes and get nervous.

Generalizability in everyday life

Generalization of learning from therapy sessions can be challenging for many people. Meaningful therapeutic change is not something that happens automatically as a result of attending weekly therapy sessions for 50 minutes. Consider how to support the generalization of skills across the time in between sessions. Can generalizability be supported either through relationships (supporters, for example) or prompts such as cue cards and key rings? Create anything that is useful and makes sense to the individual.

Prompts should ideally be made collaboratively with the individual, or by their therapist if this is preferred, featuring key helpful points generated during the course of therapy. Generalizability of concepts considered within the therapeutic space can be greatly aided by between-session practices; therefore, we would urge that this is given sufficient consideration.

The Choice Point

We have already mentioned the Choice Point, developed by Dr Russ Harris (Figure 2.5). How do we use this in an adapted way? Care needs to be taken to avoid using it in a way that people may see as blaming.

Western society already tends to minimize the role that cultural and contextual factors can have on people's lives. This is exacerbated in the lives of people with intellectual disabilities, who are often already sensitive to the idea that they are deficient or failing in some way. When used clumsily, this tool may risk perpetuating that sense of failure through an interpretation that means they have done something 'wrong'.

However, when used collaboratively and sensitively, it can be a useful visual tool to formulate and summarize a person's behaviours, and to review progress. We would always incorporate into the Choice Point the systemic factors that may operate as barriers or facilitators ('away'/'towards moves').

Systemic factors (discussed in more depth in Chapter 10) can include the views and behaviours and actions of others, practical barriers that have restricted the person's opportunity to meet their needs (e.g. financial and organizational constraints for the provider or community services involved) and the person's level of control in their environment.

Earlier in this book we presented an adapted version of the Choice Point. However, for people who prefer pictorial representations, we have further adapted this into a road metaphor, similar to the 'passengers on the bus' (Figure 3.1). Using this, different elements of the journey can be compared to aspects of life; for example, roadblocks may be compared to challenges in one's journey of life. Most people are familiar with transport journeys, and this is a dynamic and fun way to explain.

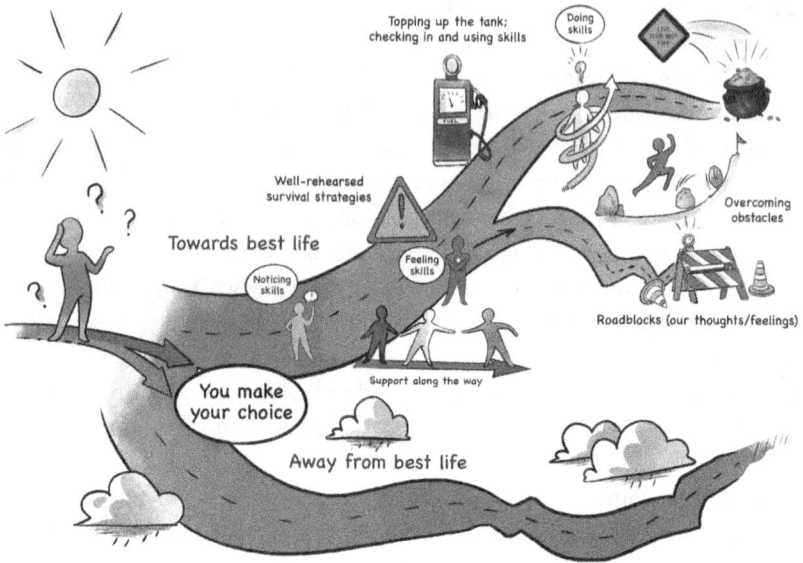

Figure 3.1 *Adapted Choice Point*

When using the Choice Point, we recommend that you devote sufficient time to first establish the person's values and goals (Chapter 5). Without a compass, a person cannot effectively start a journey and may (metaphorically) lose their way.

Once you have done this groundwork, move on to identifying the situations that trigger difficult thoughts and feelings and what the person does in response. Discuss whether this takes them towards or away from the things that truly matter to them.

It may be that you identify with someone whose 'towards moves' for their values-based goals include doing more activities to improve mood (behavioural activation), or graded exposure (gradually having increased contact with feared experiences in the service of a values-based goal). Something the person wants to do less of might include drinking alcohol as a coping method, or habitual activities used to avoid or numb the pain associated with the experience of difficult feelings. These can be explored as 'away moves'.

This 'direction' must be identified in collaboration with the person. This is challenging as some people may have difficulty considering the impact of their actions. As previously noted, diaries or visual tools can be used to encourage people to consider the links between their behaviours, their values and their goals. This helps to ensure people do not only consider the short term when thinking about whether a strategy is 'working' or not.

Doing things differently ('towards moves') includes making a conscious choice. The choice is to engage in a behaviour that may not be the instinctive first choice when managing a difficult feeling. For example, many people instinctively engage in avoidance of something that is perceived to be a threat. A person who has had difficulty with a supporter may try to stay away from them as much as possible without opening up or trying to resolve the issue. They may do this even if that means missing out on important activities. By using the Choice Point and exploring what matters most to that person, they may conclude that this constitutes an 'away move'. They might decide that a more values-based 'towards move' would be to discuss the issue with the staff member or their manager, and/or engage in the highly valued activities despite the presence of the supporter, making room for any discomfort, or to talk about the issues with the supporter. Of course, if the staff difficulties constitute neglect, abuse or a quality-of-care issue, safeguarding or complaints procedures must be considered.

You can download worksheets to use with the adapted Choice Point at https://digitalhub.jkp.com/redeem (or scan the QR code) using the voucher code UAHJYLC.

A model for adapted ACT – the Noticing, Feeling, Doing skills toolkit

We have described this as the 'Noticing, Feeling, Doing' model, which packages the ACT Hexaflex into three domains in order to be more easily understood and remembered. When the practitioner and the person are discussing the person's challenges, they can consider which parts of the ACT toolkit (the Noticing, Feeling, Doing skills) can be used to help them. This can avoid the need to use more difficult terms, such as Defusion and Self-as-Context; and having three concepts rather than the six Hexaflex elements is easier to hold in mind and recall. This model can also provide a basic framework for developing a formulation or summary of the person's strengths, struggles and values on which to build the adapted ACT intervention.

In this model:

- Noticing refers to aspects of Self-as-Context (Be Aware), Contact with the present moment (Be here now) and Defusion (Watch Your Thinking).

- Feeling refers to experiential Acceptance (Open Up) and related compassion skills.
- Doing refers to Values (Know What Matters) and Committed Action (Do What It Takes).

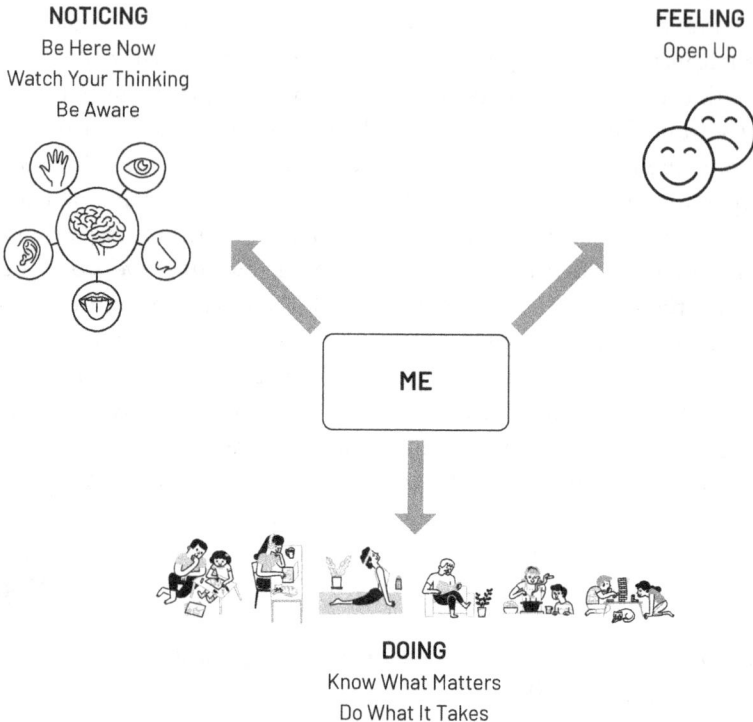

NOTICING
Be Here Now
Watch Your Thinking
Be Aware

FEELING
Open Up

ME

DOING
Know What Matters
Do What It Takes

Figure 3.2 The Noticing, Feeling, Doing toolkit

In Chapters 6, 7 and 8, we will describe each element of the Noticing, Feeling, Doing model in depth along with considering how to apply it.

SUMMARY

- We have a responsibility as practitioners working alongside people with intellectual disabilities to ensure that therapeutic approaches are suitably tailored to meet the unique needs of each individual, including consideration of cognition, language level and neurodiversity.

- It can be helpful to collaboratively develop an agenda at the start of the session to support the focus of the time together.

- Creative use of visual aids can be pivotal in enhancing the accessibility of therapeutic interventions for people with intellectual disabilities, particularly when considering abstract concepts such as metaphors, which are commonplace in ACT.

- Having a good understanding of a person's level of emotional literacy is important, along with engaging in educative work in this area if needed.

- Action-oriented experiential approaches can be useful methods to convey ACT concepts.

- Meaningful involvement of supporters, whether family, carers or paid staff, is of utmost importance when it is possible.

- The Adapted Choice Point offers a visual formulation tool that can be used to collaboratively identify actions that are in accordance with individual values ('towards moves') and those that move a person away from their values ('away moves') (Harris, 2019).

Chapter 4

SETTING UP THE THERAPY

In this chapter we provide a roadmap for setting up a therapeutic partnership in an accessible way. We discuss issues around informed consent, power, involvement of supporters, assessment of appropriateness, and readiness for and ability to engage in therapy.

Considering the appropriateness of therapy: Who needs to change?

We recognize that some people with intellectual disabilities live impoverished lives, and that therapy alone is not an answer to that (or in some cases it is not appropriate at all). What may be needed is an approach to considering what a good life would look like at a *systems level*, but in a person-centred way (and with the person's input as much as is feasible). In other words, what can the network of support do differently, taking into consideration the person's values and needs? We believe that ACT provides an excellent framework to achieve this, as discussed in Chapter 10. As previously noted, it is essential to be alert to and assess for any tendency to locate 'the problem' within the person, when in fact the need for change may lie, or may be more appropriate to consider, within the wider system. It is unethical to proceed in direct therapy if it is the support network who need to adapt their practice. Even where individual therapy is deemed appropriate, issues will often be raised by the person that require a systemic intervention in addition to areas that can be addressed with the person. Here, the challenge for the practitioner is how to support the person in addressing systemic change in the most empowering way, without being an additional person 'doing to' them.

As we have said, people with an intellectual disability are sometimes brought to therapy by supporters without fully understanding why or what therapy is. Anxiety within the person can be high, as some people are fearful that they are being brought to a professional because they have done something wrong, or that they are considered broken and are going to be 'fixed' in some way.

People who have never engaged in therapy before, but are open to the idea of doing so, may still have no idea what to expect. Where therapy could be useful, it is important to help the person to understand the therapeutic process, and work towards alleviating fears through building up rapport and, hopefully, creating the beginnings of an effective and equal partnership.

The initial assessment should seek to establish both systemic and individual factors contributing to any difficulties, such as those discussed in Chapter 3. Initial assessments involve not only the first session itself. They also encompass gathering information from a variety of sources, directly from the person and through information from supporters, other professionals and historical records.

This initial information will support planning around where the focus of your intervention should be. Make every effort to protect the person from engaging in therapy inappropriately, being (or feeling) blamed or feeling any pressure to be 'fixed'.

CASE STUDY: Stan

A referral for therapy was received for Stan, who was living with his partner Ollie and his family. Stan was referred to Psychology Services by his GP as he had been experiencing financial, physical and emotional abuse. On assessment, it was concluded that his distress was entirely appropriate and to be expected given his situation, and that he lacked the ability to keep himself safe. What he needed was not therapy, but external support and access to relevant services. A safeguarding referral was made. Stan was allocated a social worker who supported him in changing his living situation.

Engaging Stan in therapy would have been unethical at that time. Whilst therapy can be a vehicle for helping people to explore their life situations and empower them to make changes, it was clear in Stan's situation that he was vulnerable. Therefore, there was an onus on services to step in and support. However, therapy could be revisited in future once his immediate safety and support needs were resolved.

When to intervene therapeutically – equity and ethics

Most practitioners will already be aware of Maslow's hierarchy of needs (1943), a theory of human motivations. The central tenet of this theory is that everyone has needs that can be considered as a hierarchy, represented by a pyramid. At the bottom of the pyramid are our most basic requirements: food, water and sleep. As someone progresses up the hierarchy, each tier represents a developmental level with corresponding needs. Once our basic needs have been met, safety needs emerge, followed by social motives (our need for belonging and affection). This is followed by esteem needs, our need for recognition and self-respect, and finally the ultimate goal of self-actualization, defined as

> the tendency for a person to become actualized in what they are potentially. This tendency might be phrased as the desire to become more and more what one idiosyncratically is, to become everything that one is capable of becoming. (Maslow & Lewis, 1987)

Less well known is that Maslow later expanded his model with a sixth level to encompass transcendent experiences (or 'metaneeds', i.e. the need to pursue intrinsic values that transcend self-interest, beyond the need to self-actualize). This attention to values is of course consistent with ACT. Further, Maslow never intended the model to be a prescriptive one whereby people have to achieve lower needs in order to move to higher levels. Rather, the model is descriptive and was intended to be dynamic and flexible.

Maslow's ideas remain important and are relevant to practitioner decision-making over when a person with intellectual disabilities should be offered therapy. Whilst we would advocate flexibility in its application (as with Maslow's model), we provide a Therapy Enablers Checklist (see box) to help the clinician and the person themselves to consider both basic lifestyle factors that will affect mental wellbeing and whether sufficient attention has been given to basic elements of living to enable therapy to be effective.

Consistent with Maslow, there is some degree of hierarchy. The factors that we consider to be the most important are at the top of the list.

Therapy Enablers Checklist

- Stable accommodation
- Stable physical health
- Having access to appropriate levels of support in daily life
- Having structured and personally meaningful activities
- A reasonable sleeping routine
- Having opportunities to make choices about life decisions
- Some level of exercise and basic elements of a healthy diet
- Having social connections aside from paid supporters

Many people with an intellectual disability are not fortunate enough to have a life situation that is likely to bring about or support good mental health, and without the correct support in place, some people may struggle with talking therapies, so it is especially important to ensure that key basic elements comprising quality of life are in place to a sufficient degree when deciding whether therapy is indicated. Someone in an extremely chaotic life situation with very poor physical health is unlikely to be able to engage in psychological therapy, and these issues may need to be addressed in the first instance. For practitioners working in teams, the first objective may be to support the person to achieve a stable base by involving and consulting with other professionals. It may be that the practitioner and the person decide, for example, that a support package needs to be put in place or amended, which may completely resolve the person's distress. Or it may be considered that the person needs nursing support to improve physical health before considering therapy. We would not consider intervening therapeutically with someone who was in considerable treatable pain, or whose diabetes was poorly controlled to the extent that they were unwell, since such issues would make it difficult for them to engage in therapy.

A key difference when working with people with intellectual disabilities is that the practitioner, rather than the person, may have the greatest influence on deciding the appropriateness of therapy. Some people, and at times their supporters, may not recognize the inappropriateness of engaging in therapy (and nor would we expect them to, since they are not trained to assess in this area). At times, practitioners in our field can be afforded more influence than is comfortable, but it is an important responsibility to recognize. Formulation is crucial in establishing whether direct ACT intervention might be appropriate: Is the difficulty located in the individual, or are systemic factors the key influencers? Are the person's difficulties maladaptive, or rather a normal response to life events? Is this about carer discomfort with normal levels of distress (e.g. sadness at the loss of a loved one)? In essence, would a person without an intellectual disability be referred for therapy in this circumstance?

Equally, adopt flexibility and take into consideration the person's own values and capacity in making lifestyle decisions. No one should be excluding people from accessing therapy because their lives look different to ours. There may also be instances whereby some of the checklist factors are considered and addressed *through* individual therapy. The psychological flexibility of the practitioner and the individual is key in decision-making about the appropriateness of therapy.

There are times we have worked with individuals who have not had stable housing; since the speed at which accommodation is changed can be slow, it would be morally wrong to withhold therapy if the need is great. Similarly, we would not rule out working therapeutically with a person with physical health issues, such as high alcohol usage (as long as this was not occurring in session), since addressing underlying psychological issues may in fact reduce the alcohol usage. An important principle is that just as it is crucial that, as a practitioner, you do not collude with any systemic location of the problem within the person or any unrealistic expectations of therapy, it is important that people with intellectual disabilities are afforded the same opportunities as anyone else. We would not exclude a person without an intellectual disability from therapy if they were socially isolated or struggling with their health and this was impacting upon their psychological wellbeing. The caveat is that, for some people with intellectual disabilities, the wider system rather than the person has the power to make the necessary changes. The key element is the use of clinical judgement based on good formulation about where change is needed, and the degree to which *sufficient*, rather than all, of the enabling basic lifestyle factors are in place. Just as Maslow never actually proposed that higher level needs could only be met once lower ones had been achieved, we do not propose a prescriptive approach to considering the presence of enablers of therapy.

Goals

ACT focuses on developing behavioural values-based goals that are established through specific structured exercises and guided exploration. Ideally these should be 'SMART' goals, that is:

- **S**pecific: What do you want to accomplish?
- **M**easurable: How can progress be measured?
- **A**chievable: Is it realistically possible to achieve the goal? What steps need to be taken?
- **R**elevant: Does this goal align with my values? Why do I want to achieve this goal?
- **T**imely: How long might it take to achieve this goal? Do I have a realistic time frame in mind?

This approach can be extremely useful for someone with an intellectual disability who may struggle with open questions and may not initially know what it is they would like to change. Alternatively, some people know what areas of life they feel unhappy with but due to a lack of empowerment struggle to imagine change. As we have said, the development of values-based goals might not take place in the early part of therapy; it may take time. The person may need the process of therapy itself to become in tune with and confident in stating what matters to them and in being supported and encouraged to imagine and think possible a different future. For many people with intellectual disabilities, self-individuation (a psychoanalytical term that describes the process by which we can fulfil our potential) has not occurred. Therapy can be the place where this process begins.

We have developed a variety of easy-read versions of values/goals exercises that can be used in early therapy sessions and reviewed in later ones, which you can download at https://digitalhub.jkp.com/redeem (or scan the QR code) using the voucher code UAHJYLC.

It may not be possible to establish detailed goals until values have been explored. However, in some cases people may already have some idea of their goals, although this may be subject to review following values work (and may often help to guide that values work). Take care to explore *whose* goals the person is describing and do your best to gauge whether they appear to be something that truly matters to them.

Some therapy services will make a lack of clear goals an exclusion criterion. Although we understand the need to feel confident that the person has an idea of what areas in life they wish to change, many people with intellectual disabilities can, as we have said, struggle in this area. A strength of ACT is that the process itself facilitates people to begin to identify their values-based goals. When we engage in therapy with people with intellectual disabilities, we do not expect people to know these from the start.

The goals and values elements of ACT can be used as a standalone piece of work to help the person become more in tune with what matters to them and what they want in life.

For people who come to therapy with goals, it is common (and understandable) for people to state they want to 'feel less anxiety' or 'feel happier'. These are emotional goals, consistent with an agenda of emotional control. No one should be criticized for this. It is normal to want to reduce distress. Some services even have a strong focus on the reduction of 'symptoms'.

However, Russ Harris describes these as 'dead person's goals'; such goals are, in other words, things that a dead person could always do better than a living person, such as not feeling anxious, sad or angry (Peterson, 2021). We do not generally advocate using this concept directly with people with intellectual disabilities, as it is likely to be difficult to understand and could cause distress. But it can help practitioners decide whether individuals need support in creating behavioural and active goals that focus on what they can do more of. Additionally, it encourages working with individuals to develop goals that are not centred on emotional control.

Who delivers the therapy?

In addition to completing a high-quality ACT course, we recommend practitioners have some understanding of how to adapt therapies to working with people with intellectual disabilities. This could be via training, reading, direct experience or consultation with intellectual disability specialists. In the UK, the Equality Act 2010 proscribes denying access to therapy on the basis of intellectual disability. At the same time, no practitioner should work beyond the realms of their competence. Therefore, it may be the case that, where someone has a more significant intellectual disability, the practitioner will need to take steps to skill themselves up and feel confident in adapting their intervention.

Consent

Informed consent is crucial, but ensuring informed consent to therapy and to using ACT specifically can be challenging, since many people are not familiar with therapy nor with different therapeutic models. Many people have not had previous therapy and most therapy models, perhaps with the exception of CBT, are not in common parlance. Someone with an intellectual disability might find this type of information difficult to comprehend and outside of the usual realms of experience or exposure. In such cases, the practitioner will need to decide whether ACT is an appropriate intervention. This decision should be based on assessment and formulation, taking account of the person's wishes and goals (where the person is aware of them) and considering the Therapy Enablers Checklist. If indicated at this point, the appropriateness and acceptability to the person can be tested out by 'giving it a go'.

Adapted leaflets and/or YouTube videos can then be used to enable discussions and maximize understanding. As with the wider population, some people attend therapy with preconceived ideas about what is involved. Some people expect they will need to 'delve into' the past. It is common for people to be advised by well-meaning supporters as to what they should discuss in a session. It can therefore be useful to explain (to the person and the wider system) that:

- ACT involves lots of practical exercises.
- ACT does not focus solely on the past (although it may be discussed if relevant and acceptable to the person).
- ACT focuses on what truly matters to the person: their passions, values and goals.

Where a person is clearly not consenting to therapy, perhaps because someone else requested it on their behalf, therapy should obviously not take place.

However, the situation is often less clear cut. Some people will make it plain that they do not wish to engage in therapy, either saying so or 'voting with their feet' (i.e. not attending sessions); some people may 'passively consent'. If they are passively consenting, they may appear to attend willingly but perhaps not with a full understanding of therapy and actually at the wishes of someone else. On some occasions, attendance at therapy sessions may be one of the few activities for which an individual has protected time in their weekly schedule. In such cases, attendance may be motivated by factors other than a willingness or motivation to therapeutically address difficulties. Some people may attend because of attachment-influenced factors such as avoiding feeling abandoned or rejected by the practitioner. The practitioner should also be alert to consent and engagement issues throughout sessions, since some people may ultimately only appreciate what is involved by actual meaningful engagement in the sessions.

Building rapport

A person with an intellectual disability may be highly anxious when starting therapy due to fear of the unknown. This may be the case if the person has not engaged in therapy before, or even if they have. Anxiety can be greatly reduced if practitioners remember the importance of the key principles of unconditional positive regard (compassion and acceptance), congruence (being self-aware, genuine and authentic) and empathy (ability to understand the other person's experience). All of these are known to be extremely important conditions for the therapeutic relationship to form and for change to occur (Rogers, 1957), but they also help a person with an intellectual disability to feel safe and secure in what may be a potentially intimidating and new situation.

We have summarized five important factors that we believe are essential for people with intellectual disabilities to be able to make use of the therapeutic space. The onus is on the practitioner to create these conditions. As you can see below, there is some overlap with Rogerian principles. Specific consideration needs to be paid to ensuring the therapy has the following ingredients (which can be remembered using the acronym 'IS ACE'):

- *Informed*: Does the person know and understand about therapy, and about ACT? Do they know what to expect in advance? Do you discuss the potential (but flexible) agenda at the start of the session? Are you being open and transparent about what information others are sharing with you? Are you ensuring consent is considered at all times?

- *Safe*: Does the physical environment foster a sense of safety? Do you do what you say you are going to do? Does the person understand confidentiality (and its limits)? Does the person feel in control?

- *Accepted*: Are you using the Rogerian principles of empathy, congruence and unconditional positive regard at the heart of what you do? Are you challenging people in a Rogerian way? In other words, are you encouraging people to consider new ways of relating and acting, at the same time as showing that you wholly accept the person as they are?

- *Free to Choose*: Does the person know that they always have a choice? Do you regularly make this clear? Do you offer choices? Do you check for acquiescence?

- *Empowered*: Are you trying at all times to support the person to make changes rather than doing it for them? Are you talking to the person with the intellectual disability in the first instance?

Allow time at the start of therapy to put people at ease and listen to their story. Avoid overwhelming people with lots of information, such as descriptions of therapy tools or formulations.

Therapy with people with intellectual disabilities often takes longer, and it is important to set the right pace. Get to know the person, engage in radical listening, find out what they like and who matters to them, show them your humanity, and learn how the person best communicates and understands.

Do not underestimate the power of taking the time to truly appreciate the person's perspective, without trying to change or fix it. Without this, there is a danger of ACT being poorly received and being experienced as invalidating by the person. Without a person feeling listened to, respected and validated, one could introduce exercises too quickly that may alienate or demotivate them.

Many people with intellectual disabilities have had experiences of being disempowered and dismissed. Therefore, it is crucial that time, effort and patience is given to fostering a feeling of trust and safety before you enter into too many ACT-based discussions. The person needs to know that you are not there to tell them they have done something wrong.

The use of trauma-sensitive approaches is essential. Consider the trauma-informed principles of trust, safety, collaboration, choice and empowerment, but be mindful of the person's own trauma history and triggers. Some people may need emotion-regulation techniques before they feel able to stay within their window of tolerance when engaging with some practices. Create a safe space where the person feels accepted, just as they are.

When to use ACT

Elements of ACT can be used in a whole variety of ways. For example, it may be that you are working with the person and their wider system in a behavioural model. During the work, you identify that the person's parents are struggling with an agenda of emotional control that is inadvertently perpetuating the person's difficulties. You may choose work in an ACT-informed way (after considering consent) in order for the parents to be more able to experience and accept emotions and encourage the person with the intellectual disability to do the same.

Although ACT is a pan-diagnostic therapy (i.e. it is not tied to specific psychological difficulties), there are certain factors we consider to be indicators that make it more likely we will use it:

- The person has the cognitive and communicative capacity to engage in talking therapy.
- The person's difficulties are around unchangeable events or experiences. ACT can also be used for changeable situations, but the acceptance aspects of ACT make it particularly useful for unchangeable ones (e.g. bereavement, pain, disability or neurodivergence).
- The person is engaging in high amounts of experiential avoidance.
- The person 'buys in' to the central ideas within ACT.
- The presenting areas of difficulty fit with an ACT approach, without another model seeming more appropriate.
- There are key areas of the ACT Hexaflex that, if enhanced, could improve the person's quality of life. For example, if the person
  - struggles to be present
  - is engaged in a high degree of emotional avoidance or control
  - is struggling to have a sense of who they are and what matters to them
  - has difficulties with ruminative thoughts.

Creative hopelessness and introducing ACT

Creative hopelessness can be described as a process of letting go of what is not working (Hayes, Strosahl & Wilson, 2011). It is not used in order to make people feel hopeless. Creative hopelessness is a way to explore and acknowledge any previous strategies (usually those with an emotional control agenda) that have not worked, with a view to generating hope that there is another approach that will help the person to live a fuller life.

Creative hopelessness is not an essential component of ACT interventions. If the person comes to the therapy ready to make changes, it may not be required. However, creative hopelessness may be helpful when the person is unsure about making changes, or if they are struggling with high levels of emotional avoidance, or a high need for emotional control (Harris, 2019b). However, discussing previously used strategies and whether they have worked or not in the long term can be tricky.

Many individuals with intellectual disabilities (and lots of people without) struggle with understanding the links between their behaviours and long-term consequences. This may require some preliminary work. Additionally, shame may cause a person to find it difficult to acknowledge that what they are doing is not working. The practitioner will need to manage this carefully. Avoid engaging in creative hopelessness discussions in a way that could be perceived as invalidating, which can easily occur inadvertently. Otherwise, we run the risk of disrupting the therapeutic alliance, which we know is crucial in the success of therapy. Plenty of normalizing should be used when exploring creative hopelessness, in conjunction with an emphasis on working together in the future on some great ideas about making life better.

During the creative hopelessness stage people can be asked (with support if needed) to begin monitoring and recording their own behaviour and mood, to ascertain and help them to see the links. Supporters are often familiar with monitoring charts, but typically the person with an intellectual disability is not directly involved in using these (e.g. some behavioural assessment). In ACT, involvement with mood monitoring can help the person with an intellectual disability to develop insight into which of their behaviours are workable and which are not. It may be tempting for a practitioner to rush this part in eagerness to move on to 'action' parts of the therapy, but these self-monitoring aspects are important.

It is a considerable shift for people to move from an agenda of symptom reduction. It has also been found that monitoring one's own behaviour can in itself be effective in causing change, and creative hopelessness can be the initial step towards increased self-inquiry and monitoring. If a person concludes that previous attempts to feel better have been *understandable yet also ineffective*, it is likely they are ready to consider *willingness* as an alternative, and discuss further how ACT could potentially help.

The assessment process
Appreciation of context

Exploring context includes the exploration of both immediate and historical factors, gathered either from the person themselves, supporters or historical records. This is a vital part of the assessment process, which can be more protracted when working with someone with an intellectual disability. Establishing current contextual factors can involve anything from a formal functional analysis to an inquisitive approach at a simpler level. In Chapter 10, we describe more fully how to ensure that context is considered when working to support someone showing behaviours indicating distress or unmet need.

History taking

Understanding a person's history is important in building a therapeutic alliance, developing a formulation and having a holistic picture of the person. Wherever possible, this should be completed with the person themselves, as this can help to establish what has been remembered and what is significant for them. However, an important adaptation in the assessment stage is the need to gather assessment information from a variety of sources, as the person's recall may be limited or sometimes inadvertently inaccurate. For example, timescales can sometimes be wrong, or the person themselves may not be aware of, or recall, significant events.

Accessing the person's health, social care or educational records and speaking to supporters (with consent) can often be an important part of information gathering. This extends the assessment period but can be incredibly helpful. From this information you may be able to establish what previous therapy the person has had, and what was or was not helpful about it. This can be used to inform the current intervention plan.

Using a timeline (quite simply, a pictorial or written chronology of important events and experiences) can be a useful visual tool to explore people's life histories. Life story work can be another (Ledger et al., 2022); a life story book is a creatively developed visual (usually) narrative of a person's life, which may include significant people, events, likes/dislikes and memories. Adapted genograms (a type of family tree) and circles of support (a group of family, friends and supportive workers who come together to give support and friendship to a person) can also be helpful to gather a comprehensive picture of who is important in the person's life and in sparking off important conversations. More detail can be found in Chapter 6 in relation to Self-as-Context.

Ensure that during the assessment phase you have a good picture of the person's physical health, finances, support from others, social network and adaptive skills. You also need to be alert to any potential barriers to the person achieving their goals.

Structuring the sessions

ACT is not a prescriptive, mechanistic type of therapeutic approach. This can be a strength in terms of flexibility and person-centredness. However, there are some considerations of structure, by no means exclusive to working with people with intellectual disabilities, that can be helpful.

Talking therapy is a strange activity in many ways. Talking for an hour or so on a regular basis with the aim of the person changing areas of life outside of that hour is a concept that will be alien to many people. We must not assume that the person with an intellectual disability understands the purpose of the enterprise. It is likely to be vastly different to other experiences if it is the person's first therapy encounter.

What can be expected from both parties should be made clear. This may need to be explicitly discussed and could be aided by a therapy contract. This would typically involve a written, clear explanation of what can be expected from both parties within therapy and may include details such as frequency, homework, involvement of supporters and location.

Having some structure to the sessions can be extremely helpful. It may not be needed for everyone but is something to consider. Having a basic schedule for each session is one such approach. This can be written on a sheet or board, perhaps using visual symbols (as described in further detail in Chapter 3). Even if the person does not read, the items can be shown and read aloud and ticked off as the session progresses. These could be ticked off by the person themselves to foster a sense of collaboration and empowerment. The session may typically begin with reviewing the previous week's practice (including problem-solving for future similar scenarios), reviewing progress in terms of overall objectives, learning some new skills in session, and, as used by Jahoda et al. (2017), agreeing some practice for the next week. Ensure flexibility within this to allow for the practitioner to be alert and responsive to what comes up within the session (sometimes referred to as 'dancing around the Hexaflex'). An ACT colleague of ours, Dr Elizabeth Burnside, describes a 'three courses' approach to structuring ACT sessions, and we find this to be a really helpful rule of thumb. In this analogy, sessions are considered in three parts: starters, main courses and desserts.

- Starters consist of ways to introduce concepts, such as relevant conversations, exercises and metaphors.
- Main courses are about practising within session. Main courses often consist of exercises to give the person experience of the concepts and skills in a felt sense, not just as abstract ideas.
- Desserts are about helping the person consider how they can use ACT skills in day-to-day life, including home practice exercises. Desserts often include some aspects of Committed Action and collaborative consideration (often alongside supporters) of how this may be practically achieved after the session.

Co-constructing a roadmap for the therapy

Consistent with the analogy of a journey as introduced earlier in this book, we can consider the development of a (flexible) therapy plan as a 'roadmap' for the person's journey. Developing a therapy roadmap should be completed in a person-centred way. We must start with what the person brings: what the person is communicating verbally about what matters to them, and what they are telling us with their actions, including body language, as some people will not be able to communicate this verbally. The latter is highly important since some people can lack awareness or the confidence in their perspectives, but this information can still be (tentatively) gathered through observation of interactions. How does the person enter the room? How do they take up the space and position themselves? What are the interactions like between them and the carer? We can begin to hypothesize about values from the very start by what we see both inside and outside the therapy room (when arranging appointments, or in waiting room interactions).

In our experience, it can be useful to start with identifying people's values. One can use this both to establish and increase motivation and to develop the therapeutic alliance. If you can demonstrate that you are truly interested in what matters to the person, you can aid them in putting their trust in you, supporting them to feel that you may be able to offer something unique in their lives.

Values also act as a compass for therapy. If you do not know where you want to get to, your journey may be aimless. It may feel as though a person is taking 'many wrong turns' along the way. The case of Catherine outlined below and depicted in Figure 4.1 provides an example of this roadmap analogy used in practice, specifically tailored to individual interests.

CASE STUDY: Catherine (1) – Catching what really matters

Catherine was in her late forties and lived independently in her own flat close to the local town centre; she had been diagnosed with a mild learning disability in her early twenties. She loved dancing, musical theatre and Motown music, and had a part-time job at a local shop. Catherine had previously received psychological support from local intellectual disability services following some difficult life experiences, including the loss of close family members, which had led to low mood and had exacerbated her existing anxiety. Subsequently, Catherine was referred again for 'emotional support'. During early therapy sessions, she and the therapist collaboratively identified aspects of her current situation with which she felt she would benefit from some support. These included:

- 'Flashbacks of bad memories from the past (worse at night-time)'
- 'Panic attacks when I feel really worried'
- 'Snapping at people – going off like a volcano'(especially after a bad night)
- Ongoing grief following numerous losses in life – 'Why me? Why does it always happen to me?'

Catherine and the therapist worked together to think about the things that might be helpful to support her to continue to do the things that truly matter, despite the difficulties that she had identified. Therapy sessions included discussion of the concept of life having 'ups and downs' ('a bit like a rollercoaster') and inevitable twists and turns. Catherine personally preferred this analogy to the concept of 'moving up and down a ladder', which she had used in previous therapeutic interventions. The connotations of falling down a ladder felt like she was making backwards progress.

Considering the concept of a winding road ('the Yellow Brick Road') was preferable, where the 'pot of gold' at the end can always be in sight. Despite the inevitable twists and turns, Catherine felt reassured that she would not 'fall off' the winding Yellow Brick Road.

Because many of Catherine's worries were about difficult memories from the past, and worries about possible future eventualities, therapy focused on exploration of ways that Catherine may focus on the present moment ('be here now'), gently guiding her mind back when it wandered towards rumination of past difficult memories. By considering the 'pot of gold' at the end of the Yellow Brick Road, Catherine understood that the pot of gold was just like 'values'. While they may not be attainable in literal terms, they provided a compass direction to keep her moving forwards in a valued life direction.

By the end of therapy, Catherine understood that, although worries may never 'go away', she could always aim to *choose* how she responds to them using skills from her Noticing, Feeling, Doing toolkit.

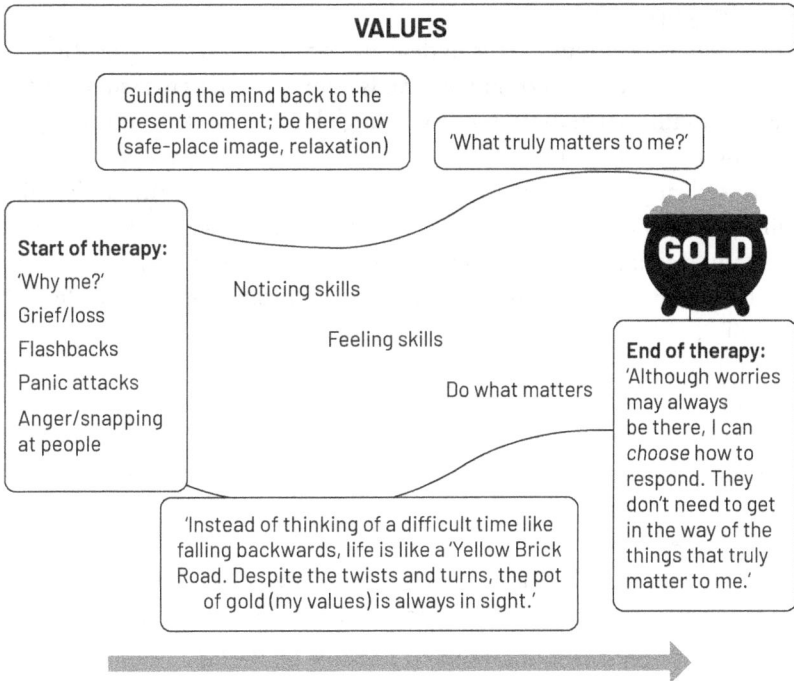

Figure 4.1 *Catherine and the Yellow Brick Road*

CASE STUDY: Jake

Jake came to therapy having difficulties with anxiety in social situations and low self-esteem. When directly asked, he struggled to identify what his goals were, or what he wanted to change. However, his description of his difficulties with socializing (negative thoughts about himself, fear of judgement), enabled identification of the values underpinning these struggles: belonging, acceptance and friendship.

Jake's poor self-esteem and anxiety meant that it was important to tread carefully in therapy to avoid perpetuating his sense of failure, and so early sessions focused on increasing motivation and instilling hope through discussion about values work. Over time, these were shaped into measurable, behavioural goals. We agreed that our plan would be to focus on commitment to these goals whilst exploring barriers to achieving them. As sessions continued, and Jake felt more able to open up in therapy, he disclosed some deeper-seated shame around his intellectual disabilities and associated aspects of his physical appearance, which necessitated acceptance-based approaches. This had not been part of the initial 'roadmap' but became apparent as sessions continued.

Building up to ACT

Some people have only a basic understanding of the words for emotions or how to identify them. A common error is for practitioners to assume a basic understanding of concepts, thereby 'losing' the person when embarking on therapy, engaging in a simply superficial dialogue about emotional experience. A clear profile of the person's understanding of the various domains will aid session planning. Some people may only struggle with particular elements and it is important to establish which elements they are.

It is common for people with intellectual disabilities to struggle with identifying thoughts, because of their abstract nature. This may be an area for more focused attention. It may be that some people require adaptation throughout the therapy. Take the example of a person with intellectual disabilities who, even after preparatory sessions, continues to struggle with the thought domain. They may benefit from less Defusion work and a greater emphasis on behavioural goals.

If, however, the thought domain is considered to be a skill that has the potential to be taught, the preparatory work would continue until understanding was achieved, and Defusion could be included within the sessions. It might not be necessary to complete all of the preparatory work at the start, as it could be interwoven into various parts of the therapy.

Some people are very capable of identifying their thoughts. Indeed, cognitions may be the dominant domain for therapeutic focus, for example in someone who ruminates a lot. Others struggle more with the emotional domain, and the identifying and labelling of emotions may require the most focus.

Assessing ability to engage in therapy

As part of determining whether individual therapy is appropriate and indicated, it is important to assess whether the person has the cognitive ability and emotional literacy skills to engage. One way to do this is through the use of structured assessment tools. The previously mentioned assessment tools described in Oathamshaw and Haddock (2006) can be useful here.

Two specific areas that will be important to assess when using ACT are:

- abstract thinking ability
- imaginative ability.

Abstract thinking ability

Since ACT is a therapy that makes frequent use of metaphor, it will be important to assess the person's ability to think abstractly, probably more so than for other therapies. Analysing the profile of anyone who has had previous formal intellectual assessments, such as IQ assessments, can give an indication of the person's understanding of abstract concepts. This should be done using advice from an appropriately qualified psychologist. Alternatively, abstract thinking can be assessed within therapy by trying out metaphors in the therapy room and checking understanding.

> The person could be shown an object, for example a ball or a plant. They are then asked to think of uses for the object other than the primary one. If a person is able to do this, it gives a reasonable indication that they may understand metaphors, since this task covers the ability to think imaginatively and abstractly.

There are some people (especially autistic people) who are highly literal/concrete and who therefore struggle with metaphor, in which case it must be used judiciously, or not at all. Others may be able to understand basic metaphors that do not involve too many concepts. This can vary according to the individual.

We have worked with people with intellectual disabilities who can understand the more common metaphors ('demons on the boat', 'passengers on the bus') without difficulty (although visuals help with the recall element). Others, particularly autistic people, could not. Instead, they were able to understand the simpler idea of difficult thoughts/feelings as monsters, or the idea of a struggle switch.[1] The struggle switch involves only one concept and is therefore easier to hold in mind.

Imaginative ability

Establish how much the person can imagine scenarios and in which modality they do so best. Imaginative ability is needed for many exercises in ACT, although it is not essential as they can be omitted. You will need to clarify whether exercises relying on imagination will be useful to incorporate into sessions in a meaningful way.

Although imaginative ability can be assessed by 'trial and error', it can sometimes be difficult to tease out which element of an exercise is causing

---

1   The 'struggle switch' metaphor is used by Harris (2019a) to describe acceptance versus resistance to uncontrollable situations and unwanted thoughts and feelings, in terms of a switch that can be turned on (struggle switch is on, i.e. the person is resisting) or off (struggle switch is off, i.e. the person is accepting what is there).

difficulty. In such cases, it can be useful to specifically assess imaginative ability with an exercise such as:

Ask the person to imagine a red ball, then imagine it changing colour/ shape. Then ask them to imagine hearing a cat miaow and changing the volume. The way they respond will give some sense of the person's imaginative abilities and in which domain they work best.

Elements of an emotionally nurturing therapeutic relationship

Other factors to consider when embarking on the development of a therapeutic, emotionally nurturing relationship include a number of key features outlined below (Shackleton, 2016). The following is not an exhaustive list but a set of guiding principles to strive for if scope allows:

- establish the therapeutic space
- use concrete communications of nurture
- establish rapport in early sessions
- employ therapeutic elements
- keep process notes/clinical records
- collaborate with support staff and multidisciplinary working.

Establishing the therapeutic space

Structural and environmental factors can make a difference to therapeutic effectiveness. Where possible, it can be helpful to ensure that the same private space, away from distractions, is available to see the person at the same time each week. So far as possible, ensure that the room looks the same each week, before the person enters. Within supported living settings, this can be difficult, so some collaboration with supporters to co-ordinate this ahead of time can be a helpful strategy.

When visiting people within their own home, try to avoid conducting sessions within the bedroom space. Where possible, make efforts to meet within a communal space (without distractions). This is to ensure that individuals can maintain their bedroom as a safe and comfortable space without association with some of the difficult experiences they may have discussed during the session.

In some settings, booking the room and therapist time may need to be done well ahead of time, and communicated clearly with the relevant networks. For example, does the person have a support network who assist with weekly routine planning? If so, appointments should be factored into the planning. There should be plenty of time allowed either side of the appointment to avoid rushing back from a previous task or having an activity to go to very soon after the appointment, as this may overwhelm an individual. At the same time, this may depend on the individual's preference. Sometimes a helpful strategy for an individual following a therapy session is to spend time with a supporter doing an activity that they enjoy, perhaps walking or visiting a local café for a drink.

So far as possible, maintain an open and collaborative stance around any changes to the session schedule and provide plenty of notice of planned breaks and reassurance of return.

Concrete communications of nurture
Examples of how to communicate compassion and nurture towards the individual that you are working with may, to name a few, include:

- checking that the person is comfortable in the session space
- offering them an opportunity to choose their seat where possible
- taking their coat
- providing refreshments.

These actions communicate respect. They will help the person to feel comfortable whilst also communicating that their needs matter to you. This is all the more important for people who have had experiences of their needs being neglected and is in accordance with a trauma-informed approach of fostering a sense of safety, trust and control.

We note here that these actions need to be carefully risk-assessed where appropriate. For example, offering individuals a hot drink during a session should be in line with a person's individual care plan. In some cases, this may not be appropriate.

Establishing rapport
'Getting to know you' practical activities or assessments can be helpful to focus the session, as well as development of a 'one-page profile' (shown in Figure 5.2). The one-page profile can be for both person and therapist, and relevant members of the support network as appropriate (such as family members, carer or staff team).

Reassure people in early sessions that:

- they have a choice as to whether they attend sessions

- it is okay to choose not to embark on therapy, and there will be no consequences.

There may be issues around non-attendance in forensic settings, where attendance at therapy may be an element of a court order. In such cases, consent does not need such consideration; but rapport and engagement certainly will.

Therapeutic elements

- Use active listening and reflection to let the person know that they are being attended to.
- Be aware of the need for emotional regulation in session, especially towards the end as the session draws to a close. Consider the next steps for the person directly after the session; will they be supported by a member of staff/family/carer, or will they be alone after the session? Consider strategies that are helpful to the individual.
- Educate the person that they may feel tired after the session; encourage self-care and nurture, and helpful strategies that they may use to look after themselves after the session.

Process notes/clinical records
Write a narrative of the session as soon as possible to process the content of the session. Reviewing these monthly often reveals patterns that may not be possible to see week to week.

Collaboration with support staff and multidisciplinary working
A multidisciplinary approach to working with people with intellectual disabilities is often pivotal to meaningful change. Some liaison with staff or support networks prior to, and in between, sessions can be helpful. We can check how the person is coping with the emotional elements of sessions and support implementation of suggested strategies between sessions. Having a supporter on board who is familiar with strategies can support practice and lived experiences away from the therapy room.

Liaison with support staff is especially needed at the beginning and end of work, and at times of significant disclosures and insights.

Troubleshooting
In this section we outline some of the most common barriers we have encountered when engaging in direct therapy with people with intellectual disabilities, along with some suggested ways to overcome them.

Struggling with homework or applying therapy

The use of manuals or therapeutic materials such as those mentioned in this book lends itself well to the inclusion of supporters, with the potential for use of handouts or home tasks for reference between sessions. As we have said, the majority of people will need someone to support them with applying the learning during sessions into everyday life.

Whilst there are important processes that take place within the therapy itself, if there are practice tasks or strategies to be applied, it can be very helpful if the person has a trusted supporter who can to help to remind the person when and how to apply their learning, or to go over tasks if the person is unsure of the instructions. This can be a paid supporter or a family member. Where this is the case, it is essential to consider confidentiality issues.

Where there is a barrier to the availability or quality of such support, attention and effort may need to be paid to how support can be enhanced. If a barrier is simply accepted, it may be as though the person is being inadvertently 'set up to fail' from the outset. Enhancing support may involve further training to the support staff (since it may be that the support staff themselves do not understand the model or their role within the therapy), emphasizing the importance of their involvement, ensuring the most appropriate staff have been selected, or requesting a review of the level of support the person is receiving (as the issues you are encountering could indicate a broader issue of a lack of sufficient support). If no support staff are possible, we recommend increasing the use of visual and technological aids.

The person is struggling to understand the model

Practitioners should stay alert to difficulties with people understanding the content. Some people find it shameful to admit they have not understood, which can lead the practitioner to happily continue, not recognizing until later in therapy that the person has been having difficulty in grasping concepts and keeping up with the pace of therapy. Give people plenty of permission to say if they haven't understood and normalize this for them. Regularly check on the person's understanding and use further simplification and visual aids if needed. There are often several options available to illustrate concepts. If one does not work, try another.

If a person turns out to be highly literal, avoid using metaphors and strive to make use of concrete examples. Reassess the person's ability to use thoughts/behaviours/feelings and their links if you have doubts on the person's understanding. Supporters who know the person well can sometimes be helpful in 'translating' a concept into a format that the person understands. Consider focusing only on parts of the Hexaflex. For example,

Self-as-Context can be difficult for some people and is the most likely one to be omitted. On the other hand, Values can be used with most people.

Finally, be alert to the possibility that even if you may have thought you could use ACT at the initial assessment stage, you may need to cease if you overestimated the abilities of the person, and it is in fact too difficult for them to engage in.

The person does not appear motivated

As we have indicated, some people with intellectual disabilities are attending therapy where the request has been made by someone else. The person may have some ambivalence about engagement or may not see the need that others do. For example, we will sometimes work with people who are vulnerable to exploitation and of being taken advantage of by others. They may not have insight into this, may not see it as a particular problem, and may not see a connection with these issues and their wellbeing. This can be frustrating and concerning for those around them who do view it as problematic and as having negative consequences.

We need to ensure we are satisfied that the person is sufficiently motivated and that we are not attributing a lack of motivation to other factors (e.g. lack of understanding). Explore the possibility that lack of progress or not utilizing the between-session practices is motivation-driven. Ask the person to rate their level of motivation. This can be phrased as 'How strongly do you feel about making changes in your life (such as stopping doing something or doing more of something)?' A simple rating scale can be used. Normalize lower levels of motivation, as some people may not wish to be honest for fear of displeasing you. If the person describes lower motivation, seek to find out what is behind that. It may be a fear of failure, a lack of hope or lack of confidence. In such cases, these fears can be explored and Defusion encouraged.

We have found that engaging in values work early on in sessions can enhance motivation by enabling people to see a direct link between therapy and areas that matter to them. It is also showing the person that as a practitioner you are truly interested in what matters to them. Engaging with, or revisiting, creative hopelessness can help as well to establish if the person is struggling to move from avoidance or other ineffective but familiar strategies. Issues around consent should be rechecked too should the person seem to lack motivation.

Just as in the wider population, engaging in therapy can depend upon a whole host of factors that may impact upon motivation. The timing may not be right; the person might not be ready or at an appropriate stage in their life to consider or to make changes. The main difference is that people who have intellectual disabilities may be less likely to tell you. Therefore, you must be alert to the signs. Open up conversations that will give people the space, the words and the permission to speak up. Finally, the person may lack motivation because the therapy itself is inappropriate for their needs.

Systemic barriers

There can be a number of systemic barriers to a person progressing in therapy. A failure to recognize these can risk invalidating a person's situation and/ or mean that we offer inappropriate interventions. For example, we often work with people whose ability to achieve their goals requires some change to their care package (e.g. the number of hours or timing of the support). Input from social services may sometimes be required to resolve this. A person may be unable to form new friendships due to the shift patterns of the staff, creating difficulties in making arrangements. The intervention may involve advocating for flexibility in shift patterns to meet the person's needs.

For example, a person may wish to engage in more supported activities, but this may not be feasible due to limitations in a support package that cannot be changed. Neglecting to appreciate the 'stuckness' of the person's situation runs the risk of making unhelpful suggestions. Bear in mind that the person may not always have a good understanding of these contextual factors. You may need to establish the situation by speaking to the wider network.

Where barriers exist that cannot be overcome, it can be useful to consider with the person if there are other, more achievable goals in line with their values. We all have realities and limits to what we can do in our lives. Where these exist and are unchangeable, we must look for other opportunities for people to live full lives in line with their values.

Lack of power

Some people lack motivation or struggle in therapy due to a lack of any sense of power to make changes in their lives. This may be realistic. Many people with intellectual disabilities indeed often lack power in their lives, and many have been in abusive and traumatic situations. The unspoken work that often needs to be done is to support the person to a position of feeling and being more powerful. In Figure 4.2, we describe this as a spectrum of power, ranging from (completely) powerless to powerful. We encourage you to think about where the person sits on this spectrum at that time, and how to move the person towards a position of power within their lives. The Power Threat Meaning framework may be a useful formulation tool to further consider power (Johnstone & Boyle, 2018). Learning to exercise power and feel in control of one's life does not usually take place quickly. It is a process of shedding the consequences of one's past, learning about oneself and discovering new ways of being, through the support of a practitioner and with the aid of a strong and safe therapeutic relationship.

We believe that the ACT model is helpful in this regard. The ethos of ACT therapy being a partnership (with both practitioner and person 'being in the same boat'), the focus on person values, and the generation of hope through experiential exercises all serve to minimize power dynamics and encourage the empowerment of people in unique ways.

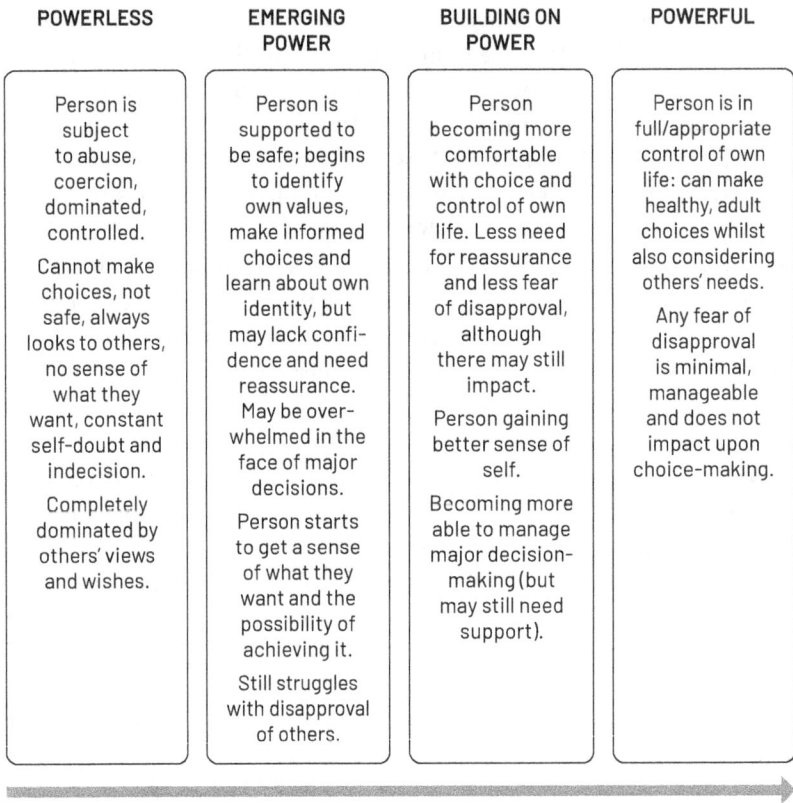

POWERLESS	EMERGING POWER	BUILDING ON POWER	POWERFUL
Person is subject to abuse, coercion, dominated, controlled. Cannot make choices, not safe, always looks to others, no sense of what they want, constant self-doubt and indecision. Completely dominated by others' views and wishes.	Person is supported to be safe; begins to identify own values, make informed choices and learn about own identity, but may lack confidence and need reassurance. May be overwhelmed in the face of major decisions. Person starts to get a sense of what they want and the possibility of achieving it. Still struggles with disapproval of others.	Person becoming more comfortable with choice and control of own life. Less need for reassurance and less fear of disapproval, although there may still impact. Person gaining better sense of self. Becoming more able to manage major decision-making (but may still need support).	Person is in full/appropriate control of own life: can make healthy, adult choices whilst also considering others' needs. Any fear of disapproval is minimal, manageable and does not impact upon choice-making.

Figure 4.2 Spectrum of power

Here, practitioner leads the person to a position of empowerment through values work, experiential exercises, formulation, developing trust, active listening, providing safe space, and generating hope and the possibility of change.

In Table 4.1 we summarize some of the more common barriers and solutions we have encountered when using ACT with people with intellectual disabilities.

Table 4.1 Barriers and solutions

Barriers	Solutions
Person cannot do homework or apply therapy.	Enlist support from support network. Bring supporters into some or all of sessions. Offer meaningful training to relevant members of the support network. Request a care assessment to review support package. Increase use of visual aids/recording of therapy to enhance recall.
Person is struggling to understand.	Simplify. Ensure assessment of prerequisite skills completed. Use visual aids. Consider if therapy appropriate.
The person is not appearing motivated.	Ask person to rate motivation (Likert scale). Use values work to enhance motivation. Creative hopelessness. Check understanding and consent. Explore fears/doubts – willingness/Defusion. Consider appropriateness of therapy.
Practical limitations – space, person's ability to get to practitioner.	Enlist supporters.
Lack of power in person's life.	Work with wider system. Use the Power Threat Meaning framework. Move towards power in therapy (Choice Point, values work).
The person is being abused or coerced.	Ensure relevant local safeguarding policies and procedures are followed. Consider safeguarding processes. Offer domestic abuse support.
Unestablished diagnoses (e.g. autism/ADHD).	Discuss with person the possibility of referral for assessment. Use appropriate diagnostic framework if appropriate.
Expectations of others.	Reflective space for the practitioner. Manage others' expectations (ideally from the outset or therapeutic input).

What can be changed and what cannot?

Time should be spent establishing areas of a person's life that can be changed, and those that likely cannot. This is very important, since without support the person may not be able to make this distinction.

Should the two areas become confused, or should the person take away a message that ACT means you should 'just put up with it', people may have the erroneous understanding that harmful or abusive situations should merely be accepted. We should highlight to people that it is never acceptable to suffer from abuse or neglect from others and that safeguarding protocols will be necessary in such situations.

Conversely there are often areas of a person's life that cannot be changed. This may be the person's disability itself, associated health conditions or the numerous traumatic events that many people have experienced. We have worked with many people who harbour feelings of anger and resentment about their disabilities, and need a space to express their rage and find ways to accept what may at the start of therapy feel intolerable.

A useful exercise can be to create a list of 'things that can be changed' and 'things that cannot be changed'. When engaging in such an exercise, be aware that you may be touching on some very painful experiences. Do not rush this exercise or inadvertently trivialize what comes up. Explore each area and the associated emotions.

We recommend that this activity is only done when a good therapeutic relationship has been formed, and you feel the person feels safe with and trusts you.

Evaluating therapy

How do we know if therapy has been effective? First and foremost:

- Is the person enjoying a more fulfilled life?
- Have they met their therapy goals?
- Are they engaging in more 'towards moves' and fewer 'away moves'?

Where possible, get the answer from their point of view or feedback. This information can be gathered from the person but may also be established via supporters too, as some people can struggle to assess their progress.

Second, the use of outcome measures can be advisable in addition to other sources of feedback. The PFQ-Ax (Psychological Flexibility Questionnaire:

Oliver, 2020) is a useful ACT-focused measure specific to people with intellectual disabilities; although currently there is no normative data there are some positive psychometrics. Alternatively, a general quality-of-life measure such as the HoNOS-LD (Roy et al., 2002) or LD-CORE (Marshall & Willoughby-Booth, 2007) may be helpful. However, it seems paradoxical to use measures of mood when the central tenet of ACT is a shift in focus from emotional control to living a life that matters, which would suggest that the focus of measures should also shift.

As well as the methods of evaluation mentioned above, it can be a helpful exercise towards the end of therapeutic sessions to reflect together on how the person felt at the start of sessions, compared to how they feel now, particularly in relation to the issues that brought them to therapy in the first place. An example of this is illustrated in Table 4.2.

Table 4.2 Feelings before and after therapy

How I felt about my worries at the start of therapy	How I feel about my worries now
'Get rid of them.' 'Make them go away.' 'Don't think about them.' 'Avoid doing the things that make me feel worried.' 'Stay at home instead.'	'I can choose how I respond to my worrying thoughts.' 'Just because I think something, doesn't make it true.' 'Worries can't stop me from doing the things that really matter to me in my heart.' 'Worries are part of being human: I don't need to let worries control me.' 'I am more than my worries.'

SUMMARY

+ There are several key areas that are important to assess at the start of therapy, and to be alert to throughout. Ensuring the person has understood is crucial, as is ensuring the person feels safe.

+ Make reasonable adjustments for neurodiversity.

+ It can be helpful to consider the role of power in the person's life, and to consider how this may relate to the therapeutic relationship. Specific attention to power can be considered via the Power Threat Meaning framework (PTM). An emergence of power may be considered a positive outcome of therapy.

- Therapy is not without its challenges. We have described some of the more common ones, with potential solutions. Key solutions are the use of visual aids and the involvement of supporters.

Chapter 5

IDENTIFYING VALUES

In this chapter, we describe the concept of Values within an adapted ACT framework. We also outline creative ways to identify individual personal values so that individuals can recognize their own values and build a values-aligned life. We discuss too how values can be used in other settings, such as with supporters, our colleagues and ourselves.

What's all this talk about values?

A central tenet of the Acceptance and Commitment Therapy model is that people experience vitality and fulfilment when their lives are lived according to their personal values. When we live in ways that are not oriented to what is meaningful, or in direct contravention to our values, we may feel listless, distressed or depressed. We will struggle to keep sight of the things that truly matter to us the most.

In some ways, this overlaps with the well-known concept of cognitive dissonance (Festinger, 1962). Cognitive dissonance can be described as 'the psychological stress or discomfort experienced when people participate in a behaviour that is inconsistent with the person's ideas, beliefs, values or environment'. High levels of dissonance have been found to be correlated with depression (Byrne, Higgins & De Vries, 2023).

Similarly, Hayes (2019) argues that losing touch with values is one of the greatest sources of psychological distress. Living life according to the things that truly matter (encapsulated by the concept of Values within the ACT model) is therefore the lynchpin of ACT. It is the driving concept within the Noticing, Feeling, Doing adapted ACT model. In our 'roadmap' analogy, values are conceptualized as the signposts that direct us on our journey, guiding us towards the things that truly matter the most, despite the inevitable twists and turns that arise along the way.

From a theoretical perspective, values are conceptualized as 'self-identified verbal constructs that confer reinforcing properties on particular behaviours in line with those values' (Hayes, Vilatte et al., 2011). In more straightforward terms, this simply means that values are basically qualities that matter to us that can act as a personal guide for how we wish to act and behave. When a person acts in ways that are consistent with these beliefs and principles it makes doing these activities feel rewarding and satisfying.

Within the Noticing, Feeling, Doing approach, values are translated into measurable goals that are met through consistent patterns of behaviour, referred to in the ACT model as 'Committed Action'. In our view, the values element of ACT can take some considerable adaptation to be accessible but is worth the effort. Engaging in values work can be very powerful for people with intellectual disabilities and their support network, providing it translates into Committed Action with which both the person and their supporters are on board.

In the UK, there is an increased emphasis on individualized care and support plans as essential aspects of supporting people with intellectual disabilities to live well, thus increasing the chance of values-driven lives. However, we know that people with intellectual disabilities can experience a sense of helplessness and disempowerment (Hatton & Emerson, 2004; Levitas & Gilson, 2001). Therefore, some people with intellectual disabilities may not know or may feel unable to communicate what matters to them. Well-intentioned people in the person's support network may have directed their lives and unwittingly influenced the person with their own values and expectations. Therefore, other people around the person may understandably form their own views on what matters to the person, yet different supporters and professionals may have different views (which can further add to confusion).

Many people with intellectual disabilities also continue to have limited options available to them. In such cases, even with an awareness of personal values, some people with intellectual disabilities may experience barriers and are less likely to be in a position for this awareness to be translated to a more meaningful, values-driven life.

While practitioners have a role in advocating for the person regarding inequalities or poor care and treatment, it is crucial that people with intellectual disabilities are supported to develop their own sense of what is important to them and self-advocate. It is often valuable to undertake this journey of discovery alongside supporters, working together to consider the factors that may enable the person to live a good life, based on these principles. In this way, the practitioner works towards empowering the person rather than being another person 'doing to' or 'doing for' the person.

There is, therefore, a strong rationale for values work and its subsequent influence.

How can we tell if someone is living according to their values?

One of ACT's co-founders, Dr Kelly Wilson, outlined some key features to be alert to that can help assess whether a person is connected to their core values (Wilson, 2009). With some adaptation, these can be very relevant for work with people with intellectual disabilities. In summarizing Wilson's principles, we can expect that a person with well-developed valuing skills:

- can freely choose actions based on what is important to them; their actions are not typically organized by rigid thoughts and evaluations about what is important to them
- is seen to get satisfaction from things they choose to spend their time doing, even when talking about difficult topics
- notices and describes a variety of behaviours that could be chosen in service of a valued direction
- can do the things that are important to them even when the outcomes are uncertain, or the situation could be difficult
- shows little evidence of judging, justifying, explaining or apologizing about things that are important to them
- usually experiences their values as helpful rather than restrictive or burdensome
- can follow a values-based life regardless of the opinions or different values of others.

In contrast, a person with less-developed values skills:

- rarely chooses direction for their own life in an active and flexible way; most valuing is described as driven by circumstances or others' points of view, and much less by personal choice
- rigidly holds beliefs about the outcomes of their actions or professes strong confusion about values
- may express hope when things are going well but rarely when things are more difficult
- easily loses sense of direction when confronted with painful events; when values are held, they are almost always held defensively and rigidly
- may resist discussions of values; and when discussing values, they typically do so only with excessive judging, justifying, explaining or apologizing (they may see values as restrictive or confusing).

Values are an important part of our work, as evidenced in the following case studies. Take Sue: she was communicating what meant most to her via self-harming:

CASE STUDY: Sue

Sue was a 35-year-old woman who lived in a supported living home. Her family wanted her to attend college and a day service, but Sue did not wish to go. The pressure that Sue experienced as a result of the family's strong wishes had exacerbated her use of self-harm (pulling her hair) and over-eating as a coping strategy. The use of values exercises was attempted but was not successful. This was due to Sue's strong desire to please, anxiety about 'getting it right' and not being sure of her values or the things that truly mattered to her in her heart.

The identification of values therefore involved being alert to them through discussion, noting areas of distress 'where there is pain there is a value' (described later in this chapter) and recognizing the topics that Sue was enthusiastic about. This suggested that purposeful activity, belonging (being part of a peer group) and dancing were important to her. The practitioner's intervention supported advocacy of Sue's wishes that were not being heard.

Plans were changed. Instead of attending the college and day service, she embarked on meaningful occupation in the form of a job in a shop. Sue loved the job and took great pride in it. Within a short space of time, Sue's frequency of hair pulling and over-eating reduced significantly, and she was able to make conscious choices to move towards the things that truly mattered to her.

Abdul was able to communicate what mattered through structured exercises and conversation in therapy sessions:

CASE STUDY: Abdul

Abdul was 35 years old and had a diagnoses of intellectual disabilities and autism. He had a special interest in photography. This was something that he had enjoyed doing from an early age when his grandpa bought him his first camera. Abdul's values were identified through conversation and use of a values card sort.[1] Some of his core values were routine, freedom and creativity.

With the help of a supported employment service, Abdul gained paid work in photography, and the positive impact upon his wellbeing was wonderful for those around him to see. This type of work fitted well with his values, as he was able to have control over his working hours and channel his creative instincts into something that allowed him financially to have more freedom in other areas of his life.

For Sarah, the adapted values exercises were helpful in motivating her to take some very brave steps:

---

1   The adapted values card sort is a series of picture cards of values, which people are asked to class as 'not important', 'a bit important' or 'very important'.

CASE STUDY: Sarah

Sarah was 19 years old and lived within a supported living setting. Sarah had epilepsy in addition to her intellectual disabilities. Sarah wanted to start going on dates but was reluctant to tell her parents due to her deep-seated awareness of their fears about her doing any activities independently. Engaging in ACT values work using simplified versions, such as the Easy-Read Bullseye (Figure 5.1), helped her to identify how much the values of independence and social connections mattered to her. Engaging in ACT exercises galvanized her into asking her staff team to help her, despite her anxiety that had stemmed from her parents' fears throughout the course of her life. To her delight, her parents were only too pleased to help, and she joined a local dating group for people with intellectual disabilities.

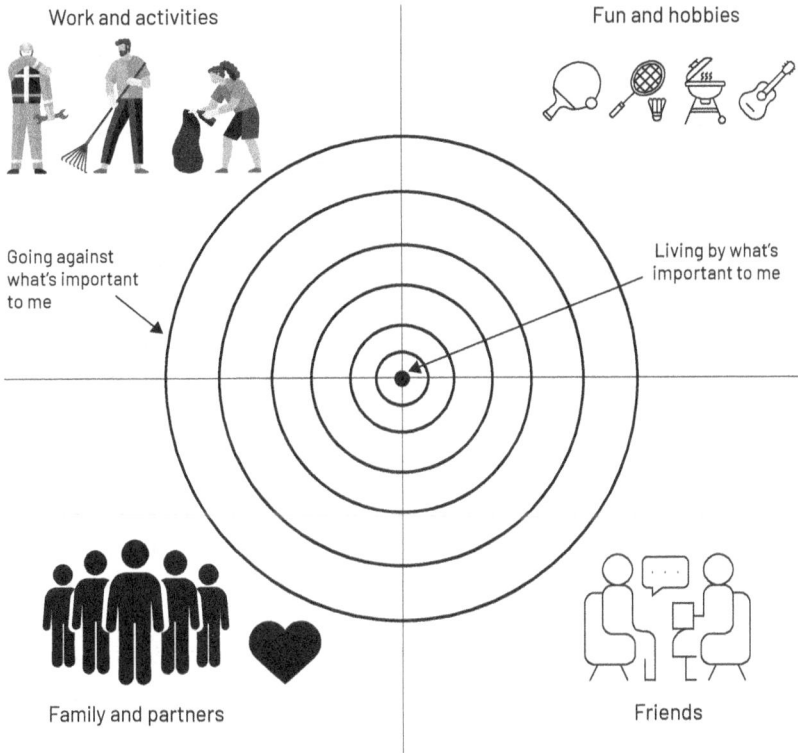

Figure 5.1 Easy-Read Bullseye

You can download the Easy-Read Bullseye worksheet shown in Figure 5.1 at https://digitalhub.jkp.com/redeem (or scan the QR code) using the voucher code UAHJYLC.

Accessible approaches to identifying values

Most people would struggle to identify their values if simply asked the question 'What are your values?' We must therefore find creative ways to support people to establish what is important to them. This may be in a more formal, structured way, or through more creative and informal methods. An informal approach may be necessary for people who struggle to identify values when directly asked, or who find it difficult to engage in practical exercises that directly explore values. Meaningful identification of values takes time and skill and often relies on creative strategies and incorporation of information from a range of sources.

Informal assessment of values

Imagine for a moment that someone you had met maybe one or two times asked you to conjure up a list of values, the things that truly mattered most to you in life; how would that feel? Would a list of values come easily to mind? Most people would find this a difficult task.

For people with intellectual disabilities, who may often struggle to verbally articulate thoughts and feelings, this can be even more daunting and tricky. Being asked to think about what truly matters the most in life may be a novel and unusual scenario. It is not uncommon within our clinical practice that when we ask members of a person's support network about the personal values of an individual they support, the response often indicates a sense of uncertainty, or that this is something that has not previously been explored in a meaningful way. However, over time, we have found ways to establish values that do not involve direct questioning.

Distress underpinned by values

Whilst there are a number of practical values exercises that can be used to good effect, we have found that some people struggle to undertake values exercises in a meaningful way. This can be due to difficulty understanding the task and/or a wish to please.

In such cases, we can look out for values via conversations about the causes of the person's distress, whether the conversations are with the person, supporter or both. We reflect back to the person our thoughts about what they have indicated matters to them, exploring this with the person rather than 'telling them'. People can explore their values via this therapeutic interaction, subsequently enhancing their sense of self.

Clinicians may also need to draw on information from other sources and carefully guide the conversation more than would be the case for someone without an intellectual disability. You could gather knowledge from family members or archived records to establish what has been important to the person in the past.

Some people have moved homes many times, and valuable information is not always communicated to new providers; the person may not be able to communicate this information. Some people may struggle with insight to establish/evaluate whether they are acting in accordance with their values in daily life. To do so requires the ability to reflect and scan through a time period to reach an evaluative conclusion.

Hayes and Lillis (2012) describe how pain and values can be considered as on either side of a coin, so that where there is pain, values can be found, and where values are present, there can be pain. In other words, if something is causing psychological distress, it is usually because it is underpinned by something that truly matters. If a person is describing difficulties and demonstrating distress through their actions, this can immediately alert you to the fact that there is at least one value there.

Values and pain can also be understood as two sides of a coin. The task is to establish what is on the other side of the coin. This is also sometimes described as the pain–value contingency.

If a person tells you they are upset because a friend turned up late to an arranged date, this may indicate that reliability is an important value. As such conversations naturally occur, you can begin to generate a list of the person's most important values. It can then be useful to narrow this down to two or three key values. With these, you can begin exploring how these identified values may later support the development of short-, medium- and longer-term goals. It is not recommended that you simply ask the person what value they are describing, since most people will not be able to answer that question.

For some people, it can be helpful to augment conversations with a suitable written or visual list of possible values. However, be alert to the possibility that even this can sometimes be difficult. They may strive to make what they perceive as the expected or 'correct' choice, possibly dependent on who is around at the time of the selections being made.

Framing the question

Framing how you ask questions about values can also be important. Many people (with or without intellectual disabilities) misunderstand what the word *values* means. Asking 'What gives you a buzz?' or 'What things or people do you love?' can be useful questions. Discussing social connections can be a helpful starting point. For example, explore who matters, who they get along with, and who they do not.

Some people may be able to consider fictional characters or famous people whom they admire and then consider the qualities they like about that person (Williams & Jones, 2022). This can also include admired people that the individual personally knows. Talking about someone they know needs some caution if that someone is a person we know well; we are also aware of their flaws and recall events when they inevitably did not act so virtuously. However, this can also provide a useful conversation about the universality of human fallibility.

For people who have special interests, which is particularly prominent for autistic people, their special interest may be a celebrity or cartoon character. Exploring what it is that they like about the person or character can tell you about their values. It can also sometimes tell you something about the type of person they want to be.

It can be helpful to explore with someone what their interests and passions are: the times and contexts in which someone feels excited and 'alive' or may experience 'flow' (which we can describe as 'times where you get lost in what you are doing' and 'times when you forget everything but the thing you are doing'). If the person cannot recall or identify any, ask the supporters to identify such times, or as a therapist, you can track a person's tone of voice and body language. Look for times, however brief, that they seem to 'light up' in conversation. You may observe notable animation when an individual talks about the things that truly matter to them.

Similarly, it can be extremely insightful to have conversations about values and the things that truly matter to a person when actually engaged in something they enjoy doing. This moves the focus away from the typical mainstream therapeutic stance of a face-to-face conversation, which may be difficult particularly for people with intellectual disabilities and/or autism. It also supports a person's ability to open up and get into the aforementioned 'flow': for example, getting creative and using felt-tips to draw out concepts as they are discussed, or perhaps going for a walk together (risk-assessed in line with individual circumstances). Such approaches are discussed in more detail in Chapter 3.

CASE STUDY: James

James was in his early twenties and was referred to the psychology department within the medium-secure setting where he had lived for the past three years. During the first therapy session, James spent 10 minutes outlining several recent grievances, which he said had underpinned a recent spate of aggression, culminating in a physical altercation with a peer. An overview of the key points of his distress are outlined below:

- James had experienced a recent bereavement of a close family member. Having been placed within a secure hospital setting many miles from home three years ago, James had lost contact with this beloved family member. Due to Covid-19 lockdown restrictions, he was unable to be supported to travel to their funeral to say his last goodbyes.

- James had recently struggled to maintain contact with his family due to difficulties with access to the telephone within the ward setting. He was particularly angry that he had not been made aware that a family member had tried to contact him and leave a message. Staff had not passed on this message to him due to an incident within another part of the ward during staff handover time.

- James had recently enrolled on a cooking course and secured a role within the hospital catering service. He was keen to learn more about healthy eating to complement the gym membership that he had been supported to embark on by the occupational therapy service at the hospital setting. However, due to severe staff shortages, James had been unable to attend the gym recently. He felt extremely frustrated to have seen peers from other wards being escorted by staff to attend the gym course that he had enrolled on.

- The same staff shortages meant that James was unable to go on his daily evening escorted trip to the ward vending machine where he would purchase his protein shake that he used to enjoy before bed while watching his favourite soap opera on television.

James's frustrations as a result of the points outlined had led to an increase in isolation, which exacerbated boredom and propensity for rumination, subsequently resulting in an episode of aggression towards a peer and a referral to the psychology department for support.

Drawing upon the content of James's detailed account of recent events, the therapist was able to derive a number of possible values. These would later be collaboratively explored with James. These served as a springboard to home in on the things that truly mattered to James. These included:

- *Family*: Sadness at the loss of beloved family member and attempts to maintain contact with family when possible.

- *Trustworthiness*: Disappointment when a staff member that he felt he could trust had been unable to pass on the message from family when they tried to call, due to an incident elsewhere on the ward.

- *Education and learning*: Keenness to develop his culinary skills and learn more about nutrition.

- *Health, fitness and nutrition*: Hopes to continue his journey of fitness within the gym setting, to complement his new role within the hospital catering service; his routine of purchasing a protein shake daily before bed from the onsite vending machine.

- *Fairness/sense of justice*: Frustration that peers had been able to attend the course that he had recently enrolled on.

- *Leisure/relaxation*: Enjoyment in keeping up to date with his favourite soap operas on television before bed in the evening.

Over the course of therapy, James was supported to consider ways that he may draw on his values as compass points that he continually moves towards, despite the challenges of the ward environment and medium-secure setting that he faced due to factors beyond his control (e.g. staff shortages). It was essential that ward staff and James's key worker team were also involved. This ensured that James was reminded of the ACT skills that had been practised within sessions at times when James may find it difficult to recall (such as when in a heightened emotional state). Examples of how James was supported to move towards some of his identified values are outlined below:

- *Family*: James was supported by staff to make a 'memory box' as a reminder of his loved one. He planted a seed of their favourite indoor house plant that he could watch grow in his room within the ward setting. James worked with staff to consider ways that he could maintain contact with family and developed a 'progress ladder' that he could review regularly in ward round.[2] This outlined the steps that he may take to move towards a visit to see family at their home, and for family to visit the secure setting for outings in the local area. James's progress ladder included monitoring of aggression, with a view to implementing effective anger management techniques to reduce its frequency. This is something that James may feel empowered to move towards now that he has a greater understanding of the things that

---

2   'Ward round' is a regular meeting (usually either weekly or monthly within secure settings) whereby multidisciplinary team members involved with an individual case meet to review client progress and discuss plans and next steps with the client. Attendees are encouraged to prepare any queries and requests prior to the ward round in order to work towards this being a truly collaborative process.

truly matter to him. This helps him understand how a choice to act in an aggressive way may move him away from (as opposed to towards) his values and the things that truly matter to him.

- *Education and learning*: James had taken a big step when he enrolled on his nutrition course, alongside a role in the catering kitchen on site at the hospital. James had a turbulent experience with childhood education and hoped to be able to turn this around. Together with staff, James identified ways that he may continue to learn and complete aspects of his course within the ward setting, when factors beyond his control, such as staff shortages, may mean that he is unable to attend the onsite education base. This included online learning and practical tasks that James could be supported to complete alongside ward staff in the ward-based kitchen. This helped James to make a choice to move towards, as opposed to away from, the things that matter to him.

- *Health, fitness and nutrition*: Similar to other values as described above, James and the therapist worked alongside his support staff team. They identified ways in which he may draw upon his values of health, fitness and nutrition within the ward-based setting when he might be unable to access the gym due to factors beyond his control. This included multidisciplinary team planning with occupational therapy. This helped to develop a repertoire of nutritional recipes that he could make on the ward, such as smoothies, and exercises that he may undertake without any equipment within the ward-based setting. In the event that he might be unable to access the vending machine in the evening, James was offered an opportunity to purchase two protein shakes each evening. He agreed to keep one for the following day. Sometimes, he asked staff to keep this in the office for him until the next evening. This supported him to resist temptation to have them both in one day.

- *Leisure/relaxation*: James's enjoyment of keeping up to date with the latest soap operas on television as a way of relaxing had been identified. James collaboratively agreed with staff that, if he wanted them to, his support team would spend time watching these with him in the evening. James valued spending time during the day chatting to staff about the latest episodes. Consideration of the topics explored during the television shows also served as a helpful way for James to talk about his own feelings, as related to different characters on the shows too.

James's story illustrates identification of values in an informal way, through identification of values from sources of distress, alongside highlighting ways in which values may become a stable base in an unpredictable world; the compass points to support onwards movement towards the things that truly matter, when other things may be beyond control.

Exceptions to the pain–value contingency

There are exceptions to the pain–value contingency. For example, a person's sensory and physical needs may be a source of distress. In fact, some people with sensory difficulties will describe their sensitivities as physically painful. However, this is a physiological matter rather than an issue relating to personal values. To confuse the two could be unhelpful.

Similarly, a person may experience distress in social situations due to sensory overload, and difficulty in engaging in activities may relate to physical health issues. This may not be reported by the person unless proactively explored by the practitioner. In such situations, the focus could be on how the person could be supported to engage in values-based activities through adaptations. The use of noise-cancelling headphones or tinted glasses may help with sensory sensitivities. For physical health issues, exploring alternative values-based activities that are less impacted by the physical restrictions can be helpful.

CASE STUDY: Tim

Tim did not want to go shopping with his supporters, and each time they tried to encourage him to do so (based on their organizational ethos of promoting independence) he would begin banging his head. Assessment of this behaviour made it clear that it was the busyness and bright lights that were distressing to him. Although one could argue that this could fit into a framework of 'pain-indicating values' in terms of a value of 'peacefulness' or 'calm', framing this in terms of a value is probably not the best way to understand Tim's sensory sensitivities, as this is really about a neurological difference rather than value.

Person-centred planning approaches

Person-centred planning tools, such as one-page profiles, can also help with the process of establishing personal values. A range of templates and guidance can be found online, such as those developed by Helen Sanderson.[3] Person-centred plans typically involve sections on the person's likes and dislikes, as well as the things that others admire about them, some interesting

---

3   www.helensandersonassociates.com

facts about the person, and how they like to be supported by others. This all gives useful indications of the person's strengths and what matters to them. When embarking on an ACT intervention, it is a good idea to find out if the person already has a person-centred plan. The plan can then be viewed and discussed. If the person does not have a person-centred plan, consider helping to develop one, or identify who else may be able to do this with the person.

We have found it useful to develop our own one-page profiles which we share with people when appropriate in the early stages of getting to know each other as part of the therapeutic process. An example of this can be seen in Figure 5.2.

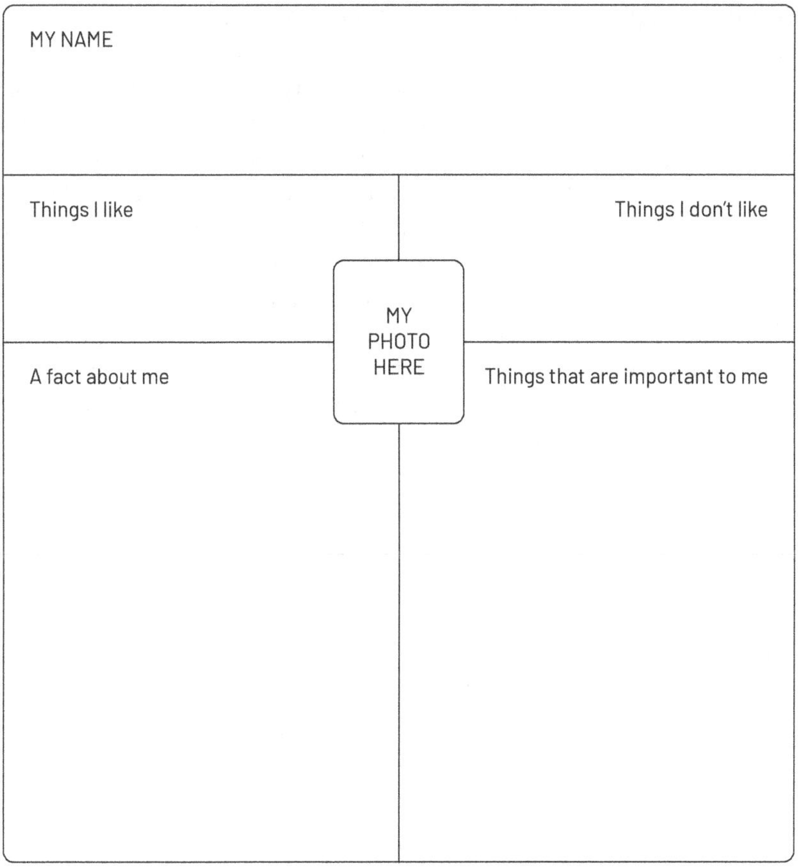

Figure 5.2 Example of a one-page profile

There is great scope to develop and adapt this brief concept in many ways. You could tailor to a theme of a specific interest or add additional text boxes that may be helpful for particular situations. For example, if a person has particularly low self-esteem, it may help to include a text box containing 'things other people say about me'. Encourage members of their support network to contribute to completing the profile and generate positive statements to include.

A cautionary note: Ensure that the details included within professional one-page profiles are consistent with professional boundaries, only including information that is carefully considered as suitable to share.

You can download the one-page profile sheet shown in Figure 5.2 at https://digitalhub.jkp.com/redeem (or scan the QR code) using the voucher code UAHJYLC.

Using photographs to clarify the concept of Values

As we have mentioned, taking photographs of valued aspects of life can support people with intellectual disabilities to clarify their values (Boulton et al., 2018 2020). The use of photography can be completed as a one-off exercise or can be done as a more extensive component or standalone intervention.

Catching What Matters is a six-session, manualized, therapist-led intervention developed with the intention of enhancing accessibility of the abstract concept of Values for people with intellectual disabilities. Each session lasts around 30 minutes to an hour and incorporates a review of photographs of valued aspects of life that people have taken either independently or with support using a mobile phone in between sessions. People are supported to consider the areas that truly matter to them, how important particular values are to them, how much they may be working towards these in everyday life and ways in which they may choose to move towards their identified values. Catching What Matters includes a number of accessible resources that can support the therapeutic process and identification of personal values.[4]

Values-card sorting tasks

Accessible values-card sorting can be a helpful tool. Values cards can be purchased online, or can be purpose-made by practitioners, tailoring the selection for each individual based on what is known already.[5]

---

4   A version of this manual is available by contacting the authors at pathnorthwest@protonmail.com. The Catching What Matters intervention manual may be incorporated into sessions by practitioners to facilitate understanding of value-based concepts for people with intellectual disabilities, and may be implemented with relative ease alongside (or by) supporters or staff teams.

5   An easy-read version of the values cards can be obtained by contacting the authors at pathnorthwest@protonmail.com. The cards can be printed off and laminated for use.

The card sorting task involves the therapist and person engaging in a practical task. Pictorial values cards are shared with the person and sorted into 'very important', 'a bit important' and 'not important.' This task will support narrowing down the values that truly matter to individuals, removing the potential for assumptions, particularly from those within the support system around them.

When completing this task, you may wish to wait until trust and a sense of safety are achieved in the therapeutic relationship, so that people feel free to explore and express their own values and not those of others.

Human yearnings

ACT developer Steven Hayes (2019) has described some key yearnings that are thought to be common to all humans. These can be a useful guide, particularly when the person is struggling to identify their values. Key universal yearnings to consider include:

- *The yearning for coherence*: People have an instinctive need to understand the world around them and experience some sense of order in their lives. Clinicians should be mindful of how predictable and understandable the person's life and world is to them.

- *The yearning for competency*: People usually need to feel competent in at least some areas of their lives. Opportunities to develop and master skills of all kinds can be extremely valuable.

- *The yearning for self-directed meaning*: People benefit from a sense of having choice and control over their own lives. Clinicians can help explore further opportunities for the person to make their own choices.

- *The yearning for belonging*: We are social creatures, and we have a need to belong to different communities, groups and families. Clinicians can look to help individuals to explore new possibilities for belonging and connection.

- *The yearning for orientation*: As human beings, we make continuous efforts to feel safe and secure, not lost within our surroundings. The yearning for orientation makes sense: when we find ourselves feeling lost, our minds take shortcuts, ruminating about difficulties from the past and worrying about potential future eventualities: 'we are mired in the cognitive weeds of our minds' (Hayes, 2019, p.211). Clinicians can support individuals to redirect people towards a mindful focus on the present, being in the here and now, to support living of every day with intentional meaning and purpose.

Challenges to identifying values

Unfortunately, some people with intellectual disabilities have been conditioned to please others. Some people are so used to deferring to others that they may have internalized the values of other people: most often those of their supporters. Due to social and cognitive factors, the person may not be operating at the level of self-individuation that is typical of adulthood. Be alert to this possibility and gently check this out. It is sometimes helpful to identify values at the start of interventions; at other times, however, it may take a while to establish and may be a part of therapy itself rather than something that is established easily and quickly within early sessions.

Many people will say that all values are important to them (for fear of 'getting it wrong' and in the belief that values *should* matter, rather than *do* matter to them). We try to overcome this by encouraging the person to pick a 'top three' or 'top five' (if doing the full values card exercise). Even then, the person may try to guess what should be the top value or may randomly choose values. We have also had people in a group setting copy each other when identifying values, as well as experience of people appearing to understand and choosing a value, only to later ask what the word meant. In such cases, the practitioner may need to guide conversations using the knowledge you have about the person, being careful not to overly influence, and sensitively check back regarding the person's understanding. It can also be useful to ask for examples. For instance, if the person chooses health and fitness as a value, yet your knowledge of the person indicates that there is little evidence that the person values this area, gently enquire about this; point out your own observations and check out that the person is making an informed response.

Provide lots of reassurance to people that there is no right or wrong answer. Offer your own or provide examples of values that may not matter to you or someone else, even though they may matter to some people, to encourage the idea that everyone is different. Remind people that we all have our own unique paths. It is also important to discourage supporters from influencing the person's choices in individual sessions (and sometimes in being present at all), otherwise this issue can be compounded.

We know what matters – what next?

Helping people to identify their values is extremely important and useful, but not usually sufficient in itself to achieve change. In fact, it may be unethical to help people to understand what matters most and then not support them in considering how to actualize it. In the roadmap analogy, it is akin to finding the road sign to your destination, and parking by it for eternity! Once values have been identified, we would recommend highlighting them on the 'roadmap' outlined in Chapter 4 or adding to the Choice Point tool if this is being used. The next step is in considering where and how much people are living according to or against their values, as well as establishing values-based goals (covered in Chapter 4).

Once important values have been established, alongside areas where things are and are not going well, you can then focus upon those values areas and what values the person wishes to display more of in specific domains. An example of this can be found in Melanie's story:

CASE STUDY: Melanie (1)

Melanie was in her mid-fifties and lived within a residential supported-living setting with access to 24-hour staff support. She had spent many years within a stable residential setting and had recently made the transition to less-restrictive community-based living. Melanie was referred to services for support to monitor transition to her new home setting, as well as support with risk-mitigation strategies. More specifically, there had been a recent increase in Melanie's verbal and physical aggression towards staff within her home. A functional analysis of recent incidents was completed, informed by both Melanie's account and written records of events. It transpired that a frequent source of friction was Melanie's tendency to have several biscuits with her hot drinks. She seemingly enjoyed doing this, but her support staff team had significant concerns about her health and wellbeing due to her diagnosis of diabetes. Recent health checks had indicated that she could do with losing some weight.

Melanie's staff team developed a strong focus on this and, as a team, worked towards reducing biscuits by limiting her ability to make a choice as to snacks with her hot drinks.

Concerns were raised about the risks she posed to staff due to aggression (based on previous altercations centred on friction between her and staff around her decision-making about her sugar intake). Melanie was supported to work alongside a therapist to consider identification of her key core values and the things that truly mattered to her, using a values-card sorting task. Through completion of this task, it became apparent that she had little interest in her own health and fitness. This simply was not something that was important to her. Things that were important to her included regularly getting fresh air and a particular love of animals, especially dogs.

There appeared to have been a mismatch between Melanie's support team's expectations surrounding the factors that 'should' be important to her, and the things that truly mattered to her. Having identified this mismatch, Melanie and her staff team were able to adapt her weekly schedule to include more of the aspects of life that she valued.

A suggestion was made that when Melanie was making a drink in the communal kitchen, staff would advise her once about previous discussions regarding her health and wellbeing. They would then step back, giving Melanie time and space to think through her next chosen action. This would allow her to decide whether to move towards or away from something that had become increasingly important to her.

In time, Melanie herself made the decision to reduce her sugar intake, alongside doing more of the activities that truly mattered to her, such as volunteering in the local animal shelter and walking dogs from the local dogs' home.

At the end of therapeutic input, Melanie's story was shared with the staff team and house manager (alongside Melanie). She played an active role in talking through the aspects of the intervention that she felt had been helpful to her. The house manager commented that consideration of values specifically had been eye-opening. The team had not previously worked with Melanie to explore what truly mattered to her. Instead, they had been working on an assumed premise that her health and fitness must be a priority of Melanie's, due to the potential health risks. Through exploration of her wider core values, she was able to make positive changes in her life by doing more of the things that really mattered to her.

Key points from Melanie's story:

- The importance of identification of individual personal values – do these align to the values assumed about the person by the support system network?
- Effective use of a practical task using values cards to identify values that matter.
- Support to identify true values, the things that really matter, can in turn, lead to improvements in other aspects of life such as health, wellbeing and mood.
- The importance of being mindful of the need for people with intellectual disabilities to have time to process information.
- The practice of providing advice only once, and then offering space

and literally 'taking a step back' to allow Melanie to consider her own Choice Point, was effective in supporting Melanie to make her choices, and whether to make a choice that may move her towards or away from her valued life direction.

SUMMARY

* Values are aspects of life that truly matter the most. They give life vitality and meaning and offer a compass direction for how a person wants to be and live.

* As many people with intellectual disabilities may have experienced a life with limited control over important decisions and choices, values are of central importance.

* Values can be hard for people to identify, but there are many creative ways to help with this.

* Values work helps the practitioner to remain person-centred.

* Without sufficient attention to values in the practitioner's work, there will be no roadmap. A practitioner's role is to support individuals and support networks in identifying and choosing steps to move towards their own unique path in life. ACT therapists can have values conversations to help people elicit and connect with what matters to them. Therapists can also support values discovery through various accessible exercises.

* Barriers will occur in this domain, and creative solutions (as discussed) will be required.

Chapter 6

NOTICING SKILLS

In this chapter we describe a range of noticing skills that can be an important part of a person's psychological toolkit. Noticing skills can be used to counteract the tendency that people have to dwell on past issues, overly worry about possible future eventualities, or 'check out' and disengage from their moment-to-moment experience. In this connection, we sometimes also use the phrase 'be here now' – an easy way to refer to being more in the present moment.

Noticing skills draw on the following aspects of the ACT Hexaflex:

- *Contact with the Present Moment (Be Here Now)*: The present-moment aspects of ACT are about building skills to enable a person to pay attention to what is happening to them at any given moment. Present-moment work can help to slow things down and therefore help people to stay in touch with their surroundings and process accordingly. This meta-ability can be challenging for some people with intellectual disabilities. Suggested adaptations and ways to overcome the challenges often encountered are described.
- *Defusion (Watch Your Thinking)*: Defusion describes the skill of noticing thoughts and being able to 'let go' of these thoughts as they arise rather than becoming preoccupied with the content of thoughts. Since it is acknowledged that identification of thoughts can be challenging for some people, ways to make this more accessible are described.
- *Self-as-Context (Be Aware)*: Self-as-Context is often considered to be the most challenging domain to comprehend. However, there are aspects that can be used with people with intellectual disabilities. Some suggestions are discussed, in particular the use of accessible life story work.

Contact with the Present Moment (Be Here Now)

Difficulties with present-moment awareness can mean that people are disconnected from their moment-to-moment experience and may be driven to seek distraction to the detriment of their quality of life. People may feel rudderless and not in tune in their various roles and with their emotions and activities, and may spend excessive time ruminating about the past or worrying about the future.

Present-moment awareness anchors

According to Wilson (2009), a person with well-developed present-moment skills will:

- be more connected to their own current experience during conversations.
- have flexible speech tone and intonation
- show more flexible content of conversation
- use verbal and non-verbal expression more consistent with the content of what they are saying or listening to
- use speech content that contains specific details, rather than being categorical or ruminative.

In contrast, a person with less-developed skills (or unable to use their skills in context) may:

- appear disconnected with their current experience during conversations
- use speech that is not fluid but in a monotone with very little fluctuation in pace, rhythm, volume or content
- have body language and eye contact that leads to disconnection from the conversation partner
- use speech that is almost always categorical and lacking in specific and detailed content
- get stuck on certain parts of their experience and if redirected may return to the topics relatively soon.

Note that in someone with autism, the above may be indicative of associated communication difficulties rather than less-developed present-moment skills.

Approaches to fostering present-moment awareness skills

There are a range of practices that can enable a person to be more present moment-by-moment. These can be brief, practical exercises or longer meditations. Both types can be helpful in terms of improving wellbeing and facilitating engagement in values-based activities. The present-moment skills taught within ACT interventions tend to be briefer practices that are not only practised within and between sessions but can be readily deployed in daily management of different situations to support contact with the present moment, *anywhere* and *anytime*.

The present-moment aspects of ACT are often considered similar in nature to those found in mindfulness traditions and models. From an ACT perspective, mindfulness can actually be thought of as relating to most aspects of the ACT model: paying attention to the moment (Contact with the present moment); watching thoughts (Defusion); willingness to experience all aspects of awareness (Acceptance); and cultivating an observing sense of self (Self-as-Context).

Nevertheless, there is certainly cross-over between different models, in that a number of simple mindful exercises can be used to help someone develop their present-moment awareness skills. Indeed, there is an emerging body of literature around mindfulness interventions for people with intellectual disabilities, which provides encouraging signs that the related present-moment aspects of ACT can be useful for people with intellectual disabilities. For example, several studies have shown that practising bringing awareness to the soles of the feet can be helpful for a range of difficulties, including anger management, anxiety, smoking cessation and inappropriate sexual arousal (Felver et al., 2022). A number of other studies have demonstrated evidence to suggest that regular formal mindfulness meditation of different forms can result in mental health and wellbeing benefits for people with intellectual disability.

A sense of safety

For present-moment practices to be successful it is very important to foster a sense of safety (an important trauma-informed principle). People need to feel comfortable and safe to try out new practices, should they willingly choose to do so. Practitioners should also be alert to the fact that some people will be sensitive to shame. They will need much encouragement and positive feedback to engage in new practices. In addition, people also need to feel empowered to decline invitations to take part in particular exercises, as well as feeling empowered to stop the practice at any point. To ensure that a person feels confident to do this, it can be helpful to agree on a 'stop' signal together at the start of therapeutic input.

This can be done by asking them how they would like to be able to let the therapist know if they do not feel comfortable with any aspects of the therapeutic sessions. This may be that the person simply verbalizes that they wish to stop the exercise, or if this is difficult, other signals such as a simple hand raise may be useful. For those who may find this difficult, options such as providing the individual with a 'stop card' to show or point to if they wish to stop the task, or a piece of paper containing an image of their choice can also be useful. We have used images of an individual's favourite things (drawn by the individual and laminated by the practitioner) to place around the room to prompt reminders of safe-place imagery when undertaking tasks which moved the individual towards the limit of their comfort zone.

Make sure to take time to get to know the person and consider how they think and process the world.

> ## CASE STUDY: The need for trust
>
> One of us had an experience of going to see a therapist with whom, for indefinable reasons, they did not feel wholly comfortable.
>
> 'The therapist would leave extremely long silences and continued to do so despite my request for this to stop. The therapist frequently asked me to notice my body sensations. Each time this happened, I felt distress. I did not feel safe enough to let go and engage in what felt like a deeply personal experience. I communicated this, and, given that the practice did not stop, I left the therapy.'
>
> However, some people with intellectual disabilities may find it difficult to communicate what is going on for them, nor have the confidence to voice this to the practitioner. We need to be alert to the experiences of our people and curiously explore them, checking for small signs of discomfort, opening up and giving permission for questions, concerns and meaningful, genuine conversations.

Setting up and introducing present-moment skills

As with all elements of ACT, we do not recommend spending too much time *talking about* Contact with the Present Moment, as learning is best done by *doing*. However, do provide some explanation, in a manner that is aligned with each individual's communication style and level of understanding. We use visual tools to do so. It can be useful to provide visuals to outline the metaphor of training a puppy (training your mind to be present).

For some people who are able to think more abstractly, a visual of someone walking through a park can often be used to good effect. Within this metaphor, the cartoon character is depicted with a mind *full of worries* versus one with where they are *mindful of what is around them* ('mind full' or 'mindful').

Practical adaptations

Offer choices of present-moment practices wherever possible, whilst maintaining a careful balance. Strive not to overwhelm people with choices. Regardless of the specific practices chosen, there are various principles of adaptation to consider for optimizing accessibility.

Many of the following general recommendations are based on published recommendations, including Finlay and Lyons (2001), Gore and Hastings (2016), Griffith and Hastings (2014), Singh and Jackman (2017) and Williams (2015):

- Use clear, straightforward and unambiguous language.
- Communicate at a pace that is comfortable for that person.
- Make adjustments to accommodate sensory impairments and physical abilities.
- Explain the content and purpose of each session and summarize the conclusions of each session at the end.
- Work together at the start of sessions to develop a signal that the person may use, should they wish to stop the practice at any time and feel unable to verbalize this.
- Use concrete examples, visual imagery, practical demonstrations and role-play to explain concepts.
- Frequently check the person's understanding.
- Regularly check in with the person, look out for visual clues as to how the person feels during the practice and remain alert for any signs of discomfort, holding a willingness to stop the practice at any time.
- Allow sufficient time to enquire about experiences after a practice. Keep questions about the person's experience of the exercise clear and simple, and consider using body map visuals when discussing any emotions that may have arisen. Allow for 'don't know' responses – be clear that this is a perfectly good answer to give. Emphasize at the outset that there are no 'right' or 'wrong' answers and ensure that all responses are validated.

Where to start

We suggest that you start with a basic and short exercise. We like to use a mindful eating exercise, as people tend to find this enjoyable. In general, we have found that focusing on more active, experiential and simple tasks is the most helpful, such as mindful walking, mindful colouring or mindful noticing of an object inside or outside of the room.

Mindful eating

A classic but effective present-moment exercise is to use noticing skills when eating a raisin. Any food can be used here, checking out an individual's likes and dislikes. We tend to use a piece of chocolate, unless the person is diabetic. Products with a variety of textures such as Maltesers which have a chocolate outer layer and a biscuit texture inside can be particularly effective! Do check for any allergies or physical health problems first, particularly those associated with any swallowing difficulties.

Dropping anchor

Dropping anchor is a popular ACT practice developed by Dr Russ Harris (Harris, 2019a) that incorporates aspects of present-moment and acceptance skills. It uses the metaphor of a boat sheltering in harbour during a storm, dropping the anchor to steady itself (but can be used with or without this explanation).

There are various versions of the exercise. These can be adapted flexibly. Typically, the practice involves inviting the person to check in on how they are feeling in their body. They then bring awareness to their body (e.g. flexing their fingers together, moving their arms and shoulders), then engage with the world around them (e.g. noticing things they can see, hear, smell and touch). Of course, this can be adapted according to what might work best for the person. You can also give the instructions one step at a time in the session to increase accessibility. We have also sometimes referred to it as the 'Hokey Cokey exercise', summarizing it as 'in (internal experiences), out (what is around you), shake it all about (move your body)'.

Noting your own hands

Harris (2019a) describes an exercise involving the person bringing present-moment awareness to their own hand. This can begin by tracing around the outline of a hand using the pointing finger from the other hand. The person is then invited to look closely at the palms of their hands, taking in details they may not have been aware of before, and noticing any judgements (e.g. 'I don't like the lines on my hand', 'My hand is pink' or 'This exercise is weird'). The person is then invited to look and feel the back of their hand. Afterwards, the practitioner can then ask about their experiences of paying attention and noticing new things.

Movement

Movement-based present-moment practices are useful as these are readily available to call upon, since we always have our bodies with us! These can be adapted based on the person's physical abilities or challenges. Where people are able and comfortable to walk, we have encouraged people to get up and move around the room (doing it alongside the person), noticing the feeling of the floor against our feet or shoes, the feeling of movement of our legs, and the air against our skin. This exercise may particularly suit more active people who struggle to sit still for long periods. It can be a good exercise to use in a group and can also be helpful when there appears to be an energy lull.

Soles-of-the-feet meditation (Singh et al., 2011)

In this exercise, people are encouraged to think of a difficult situation, and notice the feelings that arise, followed by expanding their awareness to noticing the soles of their feet (we tend to say bottoms of the feet, as this is a more familiar term). However, we would suggest that whilst people may notice an increase in calm, this should not be the end goal. Rather, the aim should be to have a sense of the feeling being manageable.

Fun exercises

Fun exercises that are engaging can help to practise present-moment skills as well as keep the person interested. For example, you could ask the person to balance a ping-pong ball on a spoon. In a group setting they could throw a ball to each other. As such tasks require concentration, people are more likely to experience being in the present moment.

Music therapy

For people who particularly enjoy music, encouraging mindful listening to music can be therapeutic. You can also use conflicting sounds such as musical instruments/radio/voice/mobile phone tracks and concurrent attempts to concentrate on a task in hand. Bear in mind that people with auditory sensitivity may find this task aversive.

Leaves on a stream

Using a flexible and creative approach, clinicians may tailor exercises such as the 'leaves on a stream' exercise, which involves asking someone to visualize their thoughts as leaves floating down a stream, to an alternative that may be practically played out within the session. For example, the exercise can be made more literal/concrete by using a washing-up bowl full of water and placing items in the water. The items could be leaves that the practitioner/supporter and person have picked together during a mindful walking exercise. You can add thoughts written onto each leaf and watch them move around in the water. The idea here is to consider ways in which the abstract concept of Contact with the Present Moment (Be Here Now) may be made more concrete.

Of course, this depends on the therapy space and availability of such items. As an alternative, there are online videos depicting the leaves-on-a-stream exercise, or the person could be encouraged to use sticks/leaves to create drawings depicting this metaphor.

Mindful colouring

We have had positive results from the use of mindful colouring exercises. Many people seem to find this engaging and fun. The use of colour can be enjoyable for some people. Bear in mind when using this that people with additional physical disabilities may struggle with fine motor skills. Adapt the mode of colouring to suit the abilities of the individual. For example, choose from a range of methods of colouring, such as pencils, felt-tips, paint brushes, sponges – think creatively! Colouring can also be used alongside, or as an extension to, other present-moment awareness tasks. Examples are collecting craft items on a present-moment awareness walking activity, or painting on paper or fabrics using items found on the walk such as leaves, stones or twigs.

Mindfulness apps

Whilst there are several mindfulness apps available, very few are suitable for people with intellectual disabilities. Even fewer are freely available. There-fore, they should be used judiciously depending upon the abilities of your person. The ACT Companion, ACTi Coach, and ACT On It are all excellent apps, but they may not be suitable. There is also the Mindful Gnats app, which is an adapted app of mindfulness techniques that we find very use-ful. The Chilltastic app is specifically designed for adults with intellectual disabilities and is a good place to start. There is, to our mind, a gap in the market that we hope will soon be filled.

Dependent on individual skills and need, apps can be used alongside supporters as a joint venture. This simultaneously supports the skill develop-ment of supporters and fosters subsequent opportunities for role-modelling the use of ACT skills.

We will sometimes create our own recordings for people and send them to their phones. It can be helpful to hear their own therapist's voice, and the therapist can create bespoke exercises.

Application in daily life

It can be challenging for people to use present-moment skills in their every-day lives. Convey that present-moment abilities are not simply about a structured exercise that is practised once a day, although this can be very useful. It is about using these skills in everyday life. Getting into a habit of regularly using present-moment skills can be difficult, as we all know. To encourage regular practice, it may be helpful to encourage prompts from supporters or add prompts such as reminder notes around the home. Change these regularly to avoid people just getting used to and no longer noticing them.

Some people benefit from routine. Therefore, integrating present-moment awareness practices into daily routines can work, although it may take some time and perseverance for the routine to be established.

In our experience, noticing skills can be a difficult area for people with intellectual disabilities to develop and apply, for a number of reasons:

- The concept of present-moment awareness is abstract and can be difficult to grasp. As ACT practitioners, a key aspect of our work is to find creative ways for abstract concepts to be made more concrete, such as using visual aids or experiential exercises. The use of both is discussed in more detail throughout this book.

- Some people, despite practice (understandably) continue to think that the point of presence exercises is to 'feel better'. This is probably because this idea is so prevalent in society. It is often better to gently encourage and shape practice over time. Encourage the person to allow whatever experiences they notice to occur, rather than falling into a pattern of 'correcting' a person's concept of present-moment skills. In time, a person may subjectively 'feel better' as a result of dropping the struggle with thoughts, and reduction in rumination. However, it is helpful to be clear from the outset that this is not the primary aim of present-moment exercises.

- Some people do not fully engage in the activities, potentially due to avoidance of the distress that this may bring. Should this occur, it can be helpful to take time to explore this openly with people. Work through any worries they may have and ensure the person is aware that they will never need to do anything they do not feel comfortable doing. It may also be helpful to explore willingness to open up and try new approaches.

- Some people fear 'getting it wrong'. This can be a natural fear, particularly when we consider the life experiences of many people with intellectual disabilities. Offer reassurance and encouragement. Ensure that individuals are aware that there is no 'right' or 'wrong' – what matters the most is simply being open to giving things a go.

- Although breathing exercises can be useful for many people, some may find that the increased attention of breathing contributes to feelings of panic. Other present-moment approaches can be used in this case. For example, some people may prefer to focus on the sound rather than the motion of breathing. Similarly, people may have hearing or visual impairments that you need to be aware of; check with them at the start of sessions together.

As well as difficulties in understanding the concepts, some people will have specific sensory sensitivities or cognitive deficits/strengths that must be taken into account, many of which can be particularly seen in people who are also autistic. For example:

- Synaesthesia is a phenomenon that causes sensory crossovers. It is as though one sense is experienced through another, perceived together. An example may be seeing shapes when hearing music or associating a colour with a name. People with this condition can still of course use present-moment awareness, but their experience will be different to people without it. In fact, there is a commonly used meditation known as ASMR (Autonomous Sensory Meridian Response) that even seeks to elicit this experience!

- Executive functioning difficulties (mental abilities involving planning and monitoring to execute a goal, including attention, short-term memory, inhibition and problem solving) may make noticing exercises challenging, but research suggests that mindfulness practices can also reduce difficulties in these areas (Lodha & Gupta, 2022).

- Some people may have difficulties in imagination that can make some present-moment difficulties more challenging. Use of more concrete exercises (e.g. items in the room, or looking at a picture) can help.

- Difficulties with interoception may make it difficult for some people to identify their emotions.

- Some people have difficulties thinking visually (but conversely some people have an especially acute visual sense).

- Sensory sensitivities, such as over-sensitivity to sound or other difficulties with sensory processing and integration, may require adaptation and consideration in sessions. However, some people with sensory sensitivities may be adopting deliberate sensory-avoidance strategies that enable them to cope. In these scenarios, encouraging being present may not be helpful (e.g. if somewhere is too bright or noisy), if not in fact aversive, leading to sensory overload.

- Other people find one-to-one present-moment exercises too intense or anxiety-provoking (as with the author's previously mentioned example). A flexible approach to consideration of creative ways that the practice may be made more accessible to the individual is important. A supporter could be invited to join the sessions to co-learn the skill of present-moment awareness. This is something that can also support generalization of the skill between sessions.

Present-moment overview

- Present-moment skills are an important enabler of other aspects of the Hexaflex (e.g. to enable people to engage in more values-based actions).
- There is a range of practical guidance around supporting people with intellectual disabilities to engage in present-moment exercises.
- Adapted mindfulness approaches and techniques can help to develop present-moment awareness skills.
- Neurodiversity factors need to be taken into account when considering barriers to developing present moment skills.

Defusion (Watch Your Thinking)

Cognitive fusion is the phenomenon of experiencing thoughts as factual descriptions of reality. Sometimes, thoughts may not be consciously noticed as an internal verbal narrative. Defusion is the process of uncoupling or 'unhooking' from this internal narrative in order to consciously notice thoughts simply as thoughts rather than being 'fused' with the content. Defusion involves the ongoing ability to notice thoughts as they arise yet not be driven by those thoughts – responding flexibly so that thoughts do not dominate behaviour (Harris, 2019).

Defusion is one of the trickier skills to learn, or indeed to teach. This is partly because it requires an understanding of the concept of a thought – something that cannot be 'seen' and cannot be observed by anyone else.

Some people with intellectual disabilities find this difficult to imagine. In addition to understanding the abstract concept of a thought, there is then a need to be able to recognize thoughts as they arise in real time. This is further complicated by the fact that humans have evolved to have a near continuous stream of thoughts. This is perpetuated by the current digital age, in which social media infiltrates life almost constantly for some.

Our behaviour is often influenced by thoughts in quite an automatic way. Within our clinical practice, we often find that people with intellectual disabilities may indicate that actions they later regret seem to have arisen 'out of the blue'. They may not have noticed the preceding thoughts. Encouraging and practising the skill of noticing thoughts is the first step to unhooking from those thoughts (Defusion skills).

For some people, Defusion is an area that is going to be difficult. It may be pragmatic to focus on different areas instead. For others (usually people with a relatively mild intellectual disability), there are accessible approaches to support people to have a more flexible relationship with their own thoughts. These are particularly helpful for the 'sticky' thoughts (thoughts that stick around and are more likely to dominate our behaviour) that are causing distress and ultimately driving the person's behaviour in detrimental ways.

Defusion anchors

Wilson (2009) gives a clear set of behaviour 'anchors' by which to monitor the strength of a person's Defusion skills. Someone with well-developed Defusion skills will typically (again, bearing in mind some of these may not apply to someone with neurodiversity):

- experience a full range of thoughts, beliefs, emotions and evaluations without these experiences controlling their behaviour
- have flexible rather than rigid stories about themselves and the world
- rarely use very concrete language such as must/must not, should/shouldn't, always/never, right/wrong
- usually describe their experiences without judging, justifying or explaining
- approach new experiences openly and hold rules for how things should be done quite flexibly.

Someone with less-developed Defusion skills:

- has experiences of events that are coloured/limited by their judgements and emotions

- has judgements and emotions that can control the person's behaviour in a way that does not seem like a 'choice' to the person
- has beliefs about the world, the past or future, or other people that appear fixed, and they often use language such as must/must not, should/shouldn't, always/never, right/wrong
- may meet new experiences with rigid expectations, even if these rules and expectations are not consistent with the actual experiences.

These anchors can be a useful guide for clinicians to gauge progress in the development of Defusion skills during the course of therapy. The extra task in working with people with intellectual disabilities is the need to consider understanding of thoughts as both a concept *and* an experience (see below), as well as the above observations of fusion and Defusion.

The concept of thoughts

One of the most important aspects of emotional literacy to clarify prior to embarking on therapeutic work with people with intellectual disabilities is whether the person is able to grasp the abstract concept of thoughts. Some individuals with more severe intellectual disabilities may not be able to do this at all. Alternatively, they may have relatively limited language abilities and hence may also have limited internal language repertoire (although there is not always a direct correlation).

Understanding of thoughts can be explicitly assessed using 'the CBT skills assessment' tool described by Oathamshaw and Haddock (2006), based on the work of Dagan, Chadwick and Proudlove (2000). This tool includes a collection of assessments of prerequisite skills for someone with intellectual disabilities to engage in CBT. A copy of this is available from the authors on request. This can serve as a baseline from which to develop the basic skills needed for engaging in therapy, as long as you consider there is scope within the person for developing this skill.

The concept of thoughts

Initially, it can be very helpful to develop a common language for the concept of thoughts. This could be based upon the person's own description of their internal experiences or a clear description offered by the practitioner. This can be elicited by asking 'What does/did your brain (or mind) say to you about what happened?'

In the early stages, it is not unusual to spend considerable time talking to people about what thoughts are. We will sometimes describe thoughts as 'words that pop into your head', or we will do exercises involving identifying whether something is a thought or a fact. We clarify that by saying that a thought is something that may or may not be true, and a fact is something that is definitely true. We will usually spend time supporting people to develop the skill of being able to distinguish thoughts versus feelings and behaviours.

Bear in mind that some people with intellectual disabilities often vocalize their thoughts directly, literally saying thoughts out loud. This may be described by others as the person 'talking to themselves'. Really, it is just that the person may be less able to keep thoughts as internal events, something that we all do on occasion! Therefore, it is in some ways inaccurate to describe thoughts as 'words in your head', as for some people they may also be spoken aloud. We recommend adding that whilst the words may pop into your head, they can also be words that you find yourself saying to yourself. This can be normalized to reduce any sense of shame. Please note that there are also some individuals who may describe an experience of hearing voices, when in fact, on further exploration this is in fact internal dialogue.

Visual aids to enhance accessibility of concept of thoughts

Using picture cards or visual aids can help people recognize their own thinking processes. This also supports the process of making the abstract concept of thoughts more concrete. Picture cards may depict various scenarios such as:

- one person telling another person off
- a person standing on top of a high place
- a person giving a talk
- a person struggling to work out a mathematical problem.

Ask the person you are working with to generate some possible thoughts the person in each scenario may be having. However:

- Some people will only generate thoughts that they themselves would have, therefore you may need to offer some alternatives yourself.
- Other people may be literal and state that they would not be in that situation in the first place.

It will be important to emphasize and remind the person that the focus is on the person in the picture and not themselves. A helpful way of enhancing this concept is through use of 'The Blob People' resources (Wilson & Long, 2018), a reflection tool aimed at the assessment of emotions and emotional understanding, consisting of a variety of black-and-white figure drawings depicting different situations and relationships. The blob figures are essentially a basic outline of a body, depicted in a number of different positions. Often, a number of different blob characters are arranged around a basic line drawing of a tree. Conversations to elicit feelings include consideration of questions such as 'Which blob do you feel like?', 'Which blob seems the happiest?', 'Do any of the blobs confuse you?', and 'Which blob would you like to feel like?'

It can be helpful to draw out different characters and use thought bubbles to demonstrate the characters having different thoughts. This can be used for examples but also to represent the person and their own thoughts. Some people may like to use characters of special interest to depict scenarios. Some people may like to draw these out themselves; others may prefer you to do it.

A mind full of thoughts

Another variant of writing (or drawing) thoughts down on paper can be putting them inside a mocked up 'head'. We know of one example where a colleague created a papier mâché head, on which therapy group members placed slips of paper where they had written down their thoughts. They could also take out and read other people's thoughts (anonymized, and with consent). It was powerful for people to consider their own thoughts in this way, which can be a way to defuse from them. It was helpful to see the thoughts of others, many of which contained similar themes about a perceived sense of not being 'good enough' in some way. Lots of people are surprised to find that other people also experience similar tricky thoughts to themselves.

This exercise can also be effectively completed by drawing the outline of a head on a piece of paper (large flipchart paper is particularly effective) and writing or drawing thoughts on Post-it notes. The notes can then be stuck onto the image of the head shape drawn on the paper. The visual and active nature of this exercise can be helpful too for many people, as it becomes fun, engaging, and can suit the many visual learners we work with.

Examples of metaphors

Some straightforward metaphors about thoughts can be very helpful. An ACT therapist we know uses the example of human senses as an analogy to thoughts: *We often cannot change the things that our senses such as sight, sound and taste detect; these are things that we simply experience. We may be able to decide what we put in our mouth and chew, but we cannot change the taste of a certain food.*

Smells can be another good way to make this point. For example, use a potted plant or stem with a distinctive smell, such as lavender. The person has the opportunity to smell the plant. They can't choose *how* it smells but they can choose how close to get to the plant and how much they sniff the plant. Thoughts are similar: they are something that we naturally have. We can choose whether we notice them, or whether we simply let them come and go and carry on with what we want to do despite their presence.

A similar analogy involves imagining hearing a person shouting across the street when you are en route to your favourite activity. You can't easily stop the person shouting. You can shout back if you choose to, but doing so can stop you from doing what you were doing, can make you more frustrated, may divert your focus away from the activity once you arrive there and could get you into more trouble. Simply hearing the sounds but walking away might be the best option.

The same can be said of noticing thoughts and letting these pass by, whilst carrying on with the task at hand. Some people may state that they would continue to shout back or become more hostile. This may then lead to a discussion about how they are dealing with tricky thoughts and any downsides to that approach. As with any metaphor, it may be best avoided where you suspect the example could be a specific trigger for that person.

A useful, less abstract metaphor is the 'chip shop' metaphor. The aim is to highlight the difference and choice between noticing thoughts and urges and acting upon them. The therapist says something along these lines: 'Imagine you are walking past your favourite chip shop, and you smell the chips. You might really like the smell of those chips, but you don't have any money. Would you try to think of another smell? Would you try to shut the door of the chip shop? Probably you would just let the smell be there and carry on with what you were doing. You can do the same with some of the tricky thoughts you have been having'. The therapist may then say something like 'We all have thoughts coming into our mind all the time, but we can choose what to do about them.'

People can be invited to consider what they think about different songs, paintings or photographs. This can help to draw out the ability to notice what a thought is by eliciting opinions and noting that these are thoughts. It can also be useful to point out thoughts as they naturally get expressed. In a group setting, this could be made into a game, whereby group members place a thought bubble on a flipchart whenever someone expresses a thought. It is often much easier to spot, point out and work with a thought as it is expressed than try to ask a person to recall a previous thought they had.

Exercises for practising Defusion
Pushing away paper
This useful exercise is described by Russ Harris in his excellent book *ACT Made Simple* (2019a). Ask or help the person to write down a tricky thought on a medium-sized piece of paper. Then ask the person to hold the paper close to their face and describe their experience, and how well they would

be able to get on with things they want to be doing with the paper in their face. They will likely find this difficult. Then ask the person to try to push away the thoughts on the paper by holding the paper as far away from their body as possible and notice how this feels (likely quite effortful physically). Finally, ask the person to place the paper on their lap, noting that the thoughts are still there but asking them how easily they are able to get on with other things, such as talking to someone, and looking at what is going on around them.

Debrief by relating the different ways of holding the paper to different ways that they have experienced or tried to manage difficult thoughts. You can then discuss whether it might be possible to try out the equivalent of placing the paper on their knees – that is to say, the idea of having thoughts but noticing them and deciding what to do rather than being driven by thoughts.

CASE STUDY: Gerry

Gerry was in his fifties and lived independently in a community setting. Gerry had previously accessed numerous psychology sessions, particularly around bereavement and loss. Gerry had a number of worries, and he would frequently ruminate. At times, his worries would become so great that he would consider avoiding aspects of life that provided him with fulfilment, such as his paid employment at the local DIY store, and his line-dancing class.

Gerry described his worries as a character in his mind that he called 'Grouchy Pete'. Together, Gerry and the therapist developed an image of this character and printed it on a small piece of paper. In the spirit of the 'pushing away paper' exercise described above, Gerry was supported to consider ways that he may notice that the worrying thoughts were there and yet choose for them not to get in the way of his continuing to engage in the aspects of life that he valued, such as going for walks, line dancing and maintaining his employment at the local DIY store. Gerry took the piece of paper and folded it as small as he possibly could. He placed this on a shelf in his living room and kept it in the corner, as a reminder that he could choose what to do with his worrying thoughts and, despite their presence, continue to live life according to his values, choosing to move towards the things that were important to him. Gerry left his piece of paper in his living room for the duration of the remaining therapy sessions and felt proud when the therapist visited weekly to be able to say 'Grouchy Pete' (difficult thoughts) was still there, but 'I'm not letting him get in my way – he can get lost!'

There are endless ways you can practise Defusion, and the particular exercises you use may be chosen based on the person's specific learning style or their interests. However, here are a few more examples (as you can see, we prefer more visual and active Defusion exercises):

Throwing paper

A common ACT exercise involves writing thoughts down on small pieces of paper. Ideally, have around 15 pieces of paper (some can be repeats). With permission, screw up the pieces of paper. Gently toss them towards the person whilst having a conversation with them about something, for example what they are doing after the session. Increase the number of pieces of paper tossed until it becomes difficult for the person to both maintain conversation and bat the paper away.

Ask the person if they are willing to just lower their hands and let the tossed paper land wherever it happens to. Typically, people will find this much easier, and it can be a useful way to demonstrate the utility of allowing thoughts to come and go and of just being able to observe this. Remain mindful in this task of how the person is feeling and be free to name that this feels like an alien concept for the therapist to be screwing up paper and throwing it around the room during a session!

Thoughts on balloons

Write thoughts on balloons. Demonstrate how these can come and go by patting them up into the air and patting them to-and-fro above your own and person's head (with permission). Alternatively, Post-it notes with thoughts written on them may be attached to balloons that are later popped or let go. Another option is for the person to write/draw/say thoughts to the balloon as they notice them in their mind; watch the balloon and thought float away.

Check for anyone with noise sensitivity or balloon phobias before using this exercise!

Passengers on the bus

Elements of this metaphor can be applied to Defusion as an exercise; for example, encouraging the person to notice their 'angry passengers' that depict their angry thoughts, or their 'bullies on the bus' saying critical things to them.

Singing or saying the word

Asking people to sing or repeatedly say their negative thoughts aloud can be a fun and engaging way to defuse: for example, singing 'I'm stupid' to the tune of Happy Birthday.

Such exercises can help the person to temporarily become more psychologically flexible and engage in new behaviours. Due to their short-term effect, their use in daily life and not just in the therapy room is crucial.

Identifying fused stories

Many people who struggle to notice their thoughts in the moment may well have fused statements about the world or other people. Some people become stuck on the same incident or idea (or small handful of incidents and ideas), even if these happened a number of years ago. Some autistic people struggle with this when the issues in question involve others breaking particular rules. Examples include transgressions and ill-treatment in earlier life, such as unfair punishment at school or others breaking rules who then did not receive expected corrections.

By their very nature these stories can be entrenched. However, it can still be an opportunity to discuss these stories as thoughts, even if the person remains firmly wedded to their views. From an ACT perspective, such stories can be considered in terms of workability. Discuss whether getting stuck on those stories helps the person be the kind of person they want to be and be able to get on with doing the kinds of things they want to be doing. For example, if a person gets very angry about an old incident and that anger spills out into disputes in different relationships, that may well be a matter that could be focused on. Creative hopelessness strategies (discussed in Chapter 4) could be employed to good effect in this situation.

Troubleshooting

Despite adaptations, some people may not develop awareness of their thoughts and may continue to struggle to distinguish thoughts from their external reality. In such cases, it may be necessary to focus on other aspects of the Noticing, Feeling, Doing skills toolkit. For example: emotion recognition, sensitivity to bodily sensations, self-soothing skills and values-oriented actions.

Sometimes, people may have an awareness of thoughts but are attached to certain thoughts being true. If this occurs, return to workability: how well is treating these thoughts as facts working for the person in terms of the life that they wish to lead?

Resist the temptation to form a conclusion as to whether the person's thoughts are true or not. A core aspect of ACT is that we do not need to determine if a thought is irrational or not (which can sometimes be very hard to establish); rather it is a case of whether it is helpful or not – whether this thought helps the person move towards or away from their chosen valued aspects of life.

And remember, practise: practise, practise!

Defusion overview

- Many of the struggles with thoughts that people with intellectual disabilities have are similar to those of other people who do not have an intellectual disability. But there is a need to focus more on the less abstract, simpler metaphors and skill-building exercises available.
- Preparation work and psychoeducation about the concept of thoughts and how to spot them will likely be needed before progressing to the Defusion stage.
- There are numerous creative Defusion exercises, many of which can be fun. Practitioners may need to trial some different approaches to see what works best for the person.
- People with more significant cognitive challenges may not be able to engage in Defusion work but may benefit from other aspects of the ACT model.

Self-as-Context (Be Aware)

What is the 'self'?

Phrases such as 'sense of self' and 'self-aware' are now in common parlance, but it is important to be clear on what we mean by the concept of self. There are various definitions of the self. From an ACT perspective, self is understood as an integrated set of behavioural repertoires (Wilson et al., 2012) involving:

1. a conceptualized self
2. a knowing self
3. an observing self.

When using ACT an aim can be to move people away from 'self-as-*Content*' to 'self-as-*Context*', but what does this actually mean? Self-as-Context encourages a focus on the 'observing self', the aspect of ourselves that is ever present. Despite life changes, role changes, age and growth, the part of us that 'observes' has been there all along. This aspect of the ACT model encourages us to zoom in on this process and recognize that there are two distinct elements to the mind. There is the self that observes the other processes that occur, such as thoughts, stories and memories. In contrast, self-as-content is where our sense of self is dictated by content, this being any aspect of human experience – what we have learnt from our past experience, inner experiences and people in our lives.

When to use Self-as-Context

It is not always considered necessary to explicitly focus upon Self-as-Context. This is fortunate, as its abstract nature can render the concept too complex for some people to fully grasp. Harris (2013) suggests using these skills to:

- Facilitate Defusion, especially defusion from the conceptualized self.
- Facilitate Acceptance.
- Facilitate flexible Contact with the Present Moment.
- Access a stable sense of self.
- Access a transcendent sense of self.

However, facilitation of Defusion, Acceptance and flexible Contact with the Present Moment are already covered elsewhere within the ACT model. Therefore, access to a stable and transcendent sense of self are the elements enhanced specifically through the self-aspects of the ACT model. According to Harris (2013), access to a stable sense of self is paramount, although a transcendent sense of self can be useful for people who have experienced trauma. It can help to contextualize suffering as something comprehendible, can reduce negative effects via encouraging feelings of flow, and the motivational elements can reduce other drives (e.g. hedonism) (Ge & Yang, 2023).

We would propose that developing a stable sense of self is often more relevant and readily achievable for people with intellectual disabilities (although of course, we should not limit our hopes for people based on their diagnosis of intellectual disability).

People with intellectual disabilities and their experience of self

Difficulties with sense of self or rigid self-concepts are more likely in someone who has had a higher number of adverse childhood experiences or traumatic events in their lives (Yang, 2023). For people with intellectual disabilities, there is unfortunately an increased likelihood of difficulties with regard to sense of self. We were unable to find any research evidence to support this statement; rather, it comes from many years of clinical experience.

There is some evidence that people with intellectual disabilities are more prone to suggestibility (Gudjonsson & Henry, 2003), which could relate to a lack of a strong sense of self (Shackleton, 2016). They are more likely to be influenced by those around them in their views, opinions and beliefs about themselves. They are also more likely to have an unstable sense of self due to all the change and inconsistency often experienced. People with intellectual disabilities may be more likely to have internalized narratives, such as 'I am different', 'There is something wrong with me', 'I am bad', and 'I am shameful' (although people may well not use this specific language). Whilst it is important not to overgeneralize, we do meet some people who have a relatively mild intellectual disability but, for whatever reason, struggle to say anything much at all about their personality, or their strengths and weaknesses. They often repeat what others have told them (including about themselves).

People who also have autism may hold particularly rigid views on self. Rigidity in behaviour means that new experiences (that may shift self-perceptions) are less likely, and rigidity in awareness means that people may have difficulty noticing their new experiences. Alternatively, some autistic people describe a lack of sense of self due to the habit of masking their natural responses in front of others.

Some people remain dependent on a parent or other family member and have limited opportunities for independence, sometimes despite having a number of skills and abilities. This can impede the development of individuation – the natural process of an adolescent or young person developing their own identity and psychologically separating from parents/caregivers with a clear sense of self. Some people do not have the benefit of healthy and empathic support from others in childhood to support this. No wonder, then, that when we begin to ask people about their values, they often struggle to identify them.

Evaluating self-skills

Wilson (2009) suggested that a person with well-developed self-skills will typically demonstrate the following behavioural anchors:

- talking about themselves in various ways without being attached to particular identities (social role, characteristics, diagnoses, etc.)
- self-concepts that are flexible, and a sense of themselves aside from these concepts.

In contrast a person struggling with less-developed self-skills may:

- be likely to talk about themselves in very specific ways
- be attached to particular self-evaluations, roles, traits, diagnosis, etc. (e.g. 'I am a .... kind of person')
- be more swayed by others' opinions/judgements of them
- often struggle to take on different perspectives when prompted.

The conceptualized self

This is basically our 'self to the world' relational frame: a narrative based on experience that may be psychologically inflexible and with which we can become fused (e.g. 'I will always be someone who has bad luck'). This becomes a self-fulfilling prophecy, since the person may not engage in behaviours that allow new, more positive experiences to take place. Thereby the narrative around self becomes reinforced. The aim in ACT is to help people to defuse from such fused narratives and create new experiences. Deconstruction of life stories can be used here.

In this practice, people are asked to write down the narrative of an aspect, or aspects, of their life and underline the facts. They then write a different story including only the original facts and changing the subjective elements. The point is to highlight to the person that their narrative is only one explanation.

Life story work is familiar to some people with intellectual disabilities and can be a way to create narratives. They may already have books with photographs, life events and other elements. These can be a great starting point. Where you don't have ready access, usually these can be created with assistance from supporters to provide photos and other visual materials.

Some people can struggle to consider any alternative narrative. In those cases, it may be that you volunteer possible alternative explanations or ask them to pretend it is someone else's story. Again, this might be difficult for some people, in which case they will need some support.

'I can be...' statements

A typical example of someone holding a rigid view of their conceptualized self is where someone makes statements like 'I'm someone who...' or 'I'm not someone who can...'. For example, 'I'm broken', 'I'm useless', 'I'm stupid' or 'I'm not good with people' (although not all self-conceptualizations are inherently negative).

We will sometimes use an exercise whereby the person writes down self-statements that they believe are true and then ask the person to think of exceptions to that rule. If they are unable to do so, we can ask their supporters to do it (but it is much better if the person can generate exceptions). Once this has been achieved, a more balanced, nuanced and flexible statement can be generated: for example, 'Sometimes I have been... but other times I can be...'.

The knowing self

The knowing self relates to noticing the wide array of our psychological experiences (Zettle, 2016). Enhancing the knowing self serves a function of broadening one's experience to those that may be being avoided or perhaps neglected due to hyper-vigilance in other areas. Enhancing the knowing self means increased attention to all that is there and not attending to only the inner experiences that we wish to or more naturally notice. For example, a person may have a rigid conceptualized self-view of 'I am the kind of person that fails'. This may then lead to an increased noticing of failure experiences to the extent of not noticing those where they succeed.

Mindfulness practices are an especially useful way to enhance the knowing self since these can be helpful in practising noticing whatever is present. Several mindfulness practices are covered in Chapter 6 and so will not be described here. It is important to try to establish how open a person is to the full array of their inner experiences and how much psychological flexibility they have in terms of their attention to experience just as it is, especially where it relates to the person's view of themselves, and to use mindfulness practices that will enhance the knowing self.

The observing self

This can also be described as Self-as-Context. As Zettle (2016) describes, if the knowing self can be thought of as 'seeing that one sees', the observing self can be seen as 'seeing that this seeing comes from a consistent perspective'. Put more simply, knowing that what is being seen (and has been in the past) is through one's own eyes. There is overlap here with present-moment awareness. It is a transcendent sense of self, the self not being defined or tied to 'I' statements (conceptualized self), but seen from a distance, from the outside or the opposite, completely detached from any rigidity of thinking about oneself. According to Zettle (2016), it is the observing self that is being tapped into with the ACT-informed question 'If nothing got in your way, what do you want your life to have stood for?' (which is a helpful and thought-provoking question we will sometimes ask people).

The string exercise

We have used an exercise whereby we give someone a piece of string and different coloured Post-it notes. We ask the person to put good experiences, or times they have been the person they want to be, on one colour Post-it and difficult experiences, or times they have been the person they prefer not to be, on another. Then we ask them to place these on the first half of the string, representing their past. The person then stands at this point (representing the present time), with someone holding each end; or you can pin the string at one end and hold the other end.

We ask the person to look at the half with Post-it notes on and notice what that feels like to look back at these. The person is encouraged to observe the different roles and experiences they have had, and exceptions to any narratives they have developed. We then ask the person to turn to the half with no Post-it notes on, representing their future. We encourage the person to think about what might be put on there in the future. This has helped people to become less fused with rigid views of themselves and their lives and become more excited about future possibilities.

This exercise is adapted from Hayes et al.'s (1999) 'observer exercise' and is aimed at helping people transcend from fused notions of the self to a sense of a self that can, in fact, be anything it wants to be. We would also argue that the earlier referenced 'passengers on the bus' exercise video also illustrates this well and can be used with clients.

Self-as-Context overview

* Noticing skills can be developed through three elements of the Hexaflex: Contact with the Present Moment (Be Here Now), Self-as-Context (Pure Be Aware) and Defusion (Watch your thoughts).

* Although challenging, noticing skills are very important for people with intellectual disabilities, whose cognitive difficulties and neurodivergences can create challenges in this area.

* All three elements can be somewhat abstract for people with intellectual disabilities but can be taught via simplified, visual and practical exercises.

* Sense of self is an important area to develop for many people with intellectual disabilities. It can be enhanced in a variety of ways, not necessarily explicitly targeted.

See Appendix 2 for a summary of the Hexaflex in relation to noticing skills (as well as for feeling and doing skills).

Chapter 7

FEELING SKILLS

In this chapter we cover the feeling skills aspect of the toolkit, which draws from acceptance processes within the ACT model, alongside related compassion skills. A key element of this aspect is to support recognition and understanding of common emotions. This skill is fundamental to positive emotional wellbeing.

Crucially, the acceptance skills within our Noticing, Feeling, Doing toolkit involve developing the ability to 'make room' for emotions as they arise. We adopt a stance of curiosity and welcome, rather than yielding to an instinctive desire to push them away, often attempting to bury tricky stuff from the past, pretending it never happened at all. Succumbing to this desire repeatedly, over and over, means that we continue to tread the same old road, in a way that has got us to just *where we are*, perhaps not *where we want to be*. Using well-practised strategies to avoid difficult emotional experiences in this way can move us away from the things and people that truly matter in our hearts, pushing us towards a life of suffering rather than solace. The compassion elements of the Feelings tools aim to help people both to be compassionate towards themselves and to truly experience compassion to and from others. Compassion-focused approaches are considered an 'antidote' to some of the shame-related difficulties that are so prevalent for someone with intellectual disabilities (Clapton et al., 2018ab).

We have already discussed the importance of developing emotional literacy, where possible, prior to embarking on feelings work. We also need to recognize and differentiate between difficulties with emotional recognition and avoidance. This isn't always easy!

It is worth bearing in mind that if you are teaching emotional literacy, you may also encounter some avoidance (conscious or subconscious). This may take many forms, including frequent attempts to change the subject when the topic of emotions is broached (deflection). For example, a person may ask the therapist for their views rather than explore the concept themselves. In such cases, it may be beneficial to make use of a combination of education and acceptance work in tandem.

Acceptance (Open Up)

As we have noted earlier in the book, people will often go to great lengths to neutralize, avoid, numb or distract from unpleasant and aversive internal experiences. It is entirely natural for a person to seek relief and refuge from suffering – who wouldn't want that? However, attempts to avoid naturally occurring emotions can become a significant barrier to living a fulfilling, values-oriented life (Hayes, Strosahl & Wilson, 2011). For example, anxiety about trying new things can stop someone from socializing or engaging in new daytime opportunities. Feelings of guilt about a past disagreement or a fear of rejection might prevent a person from keeping in contact with a long-time friend. Suppressing angry feelings and trying to stifle and push them away may also mean that a person ends up spending lots of time and energy ruminating about particular difficult events. Trying to avoid being judged negatively because of the resulting emotions might prevent someone from asserting their rights and needs. All the while, this may move a person further away from the aspects of life that truly matter to them.

Clinging on tightly to difficult thoughts and emotions can be exhausting. By choosing to hold them lightly, loosening the struggle, one may begin to experience an increased willingness to make room for the inevitable difficulties of life, freeing them up to fully engage in all aspects of the things that truly matter – enjoying the scenery on that previously feared journey with friends, smelling the flowers on a woodland walk, having long and meaningful conversations with loved ones (without the distraction of feeling tangled up with an emotional struggle), and fully appreciating the kindness of others, rather than avoiding contact due to overwhelming fear of rejection.

CASE STUDY: Gillian

Gillian was a 35-year-old physically and intellectually disabled woman. Deep down she had some unprocessed anger about her physical and intellectual disabilities. However, these felt too painful to acknowledge, in part due to the pressure she felt to 'be good and well behaved' by those around her. By pushing away these painful feelings she became overly compliant and people-pleasing. However, the feelings did not leave. Every now and again, Gillian would erupt with rage, leaving those around her bewildered and her feeling guilty and confused.

Accepting what cannot be readily changed

People with intellectual disabilities often experience situations which they may not have chosen and which cannot be changed. This may require a focus upon various aspects of acceptance within the ACT model, working towards 'dropping the struggle' where the struggle can lead to further emotional pain and suffering.

The need to be able to move towards acceptance rather than struggle with one's circumstances *where they cannot be changed* is clear. The statement 'where they cannot be changed' is important, since practitioners may work with the person to identify where potential areas for change do exist and can work with multidisciplinary professionals to help achieve it.

This is not to say that people should *accept* bullying or other painful life events, but that a position of acceptance of such events from the past may help to support movement towards current valued aspects of life. Since ACT does not seek to replace thoughts, or aim towards positivity in the face of difficult, distressing situations, the therapeutic experience can be validating of unchangeable experiences. When working with people with intellectual disabilities who are much more likely to have had invalidating experiences, this can be a powerful intervention.

Wilson (2009) provides descriptions of well-developed and less-developed acceptance skills. As with other such descriptions we have referred to, issues of diversity should be borne in mind, such as people with alexithymia.

Acceptance anchors

Those who have well-developed acceptance skills:

- have an ability to experience the full range of emotions, with little sign of trying to change their experiences, memories, sensations, etc.
- will not usually insist that some experiences must be eliminated, or that other experiences or emotions must be sought out and experienced
- are more likely to engage openly with others, including the ACT therapist, and will not usually seem to be implicitly seeking approval or attention
- may show willingness to have unwanted internal thoughts and feelings and experience unwanted external events in service of valued living, and will often freely choose such experiences
- generally notice when they have engaged in avoidance in session, will open up to their experience independently or are reliably responsive to instruction to do so.

People with less-developed acceptance skills:

- can rarely embrace the full range of their experiences
- may often try to change their thoughts, emotions, bodily sensations, cravings or memories, and may insist that difficult internal experiences must be eliminated
- rarely engage easily and openly in sessions, and often their requests for help or care are presented less clearly, or through their actions
- may report many internal thoughts and feelings or external events that they are not willing to experience
- will rarely agree to try anything that seems difficult, without putting up a fight or merely tolerating or resigning to it, rather than fully accepting it.

Describing the concept of acceptance

The notion of acceptance can be difficult for many people, partly because it is an abstract concept. It can also at first simply seem unpalatable. People embarking on a therapeutic journey are likely to have engaged in the first place hoping to reduce (or 'get rid of' in many cases) their own suffering. The very idea of the word 'acceptance' can at first seem completely contrary to that aim.

It can also seem contrary to lots of Western cultural messages around 'quick fixes' to distress: for example, consumerism as a solution to unwanted feelings – 'Feeling down? Buy a new gadget!' Hence, the way this process is explored needs careful consideration, in terms of both accessibility and palatability.

Lots of people have developed long-standing habits of avoiding difficult emotions, memories and experiences. This may take the form of: 'bottling things up' – keeping difficult feelings inside for fear of shame or ridicule if they are shared; substance use to numb the pain of traumatic experiences; and risk-taking behaviour to avoid entrenched feelings of sadness or elicit a sense of nurture – a feeling that somebody cares.

Avoidant patterns can become well ingrained in a person's routines. They become default coping approaches of which people may initially be unaware, having engaged in this behaviour since before they can even remember. Bear in mind that such well-practised strategies to avoid emotional pain have almost always served a purpose. Curling up into a ball as small as can be and silently hiding in the bedroom wardrobe may have been a survival strategy for a terrified little boy within a home of domestic violence. The same strategy may have proven difficult and less adaptive for the little boy at 25 years old and six foot tall.

Some people may benefit from creative hopelessness strategies to help build motivation for acceptance. It can also be helpful to emphasize that acceptance strategies are about 'living a good life and being able to experience hard feelings but still being able to do all the things you would like to be doing'.

We find it helpful to describe acceptance in more accessible terms, something along the following lines:

Life will always have ups and downs. Having lots of different feelings is part of what makes us human. Without feeling sad we find it difficult to know when we feel happy; without feeling scared, how would we know when we feel calm? Being able to make room for difficult feelings when they come up can be helpful, even if we really don't want them to be there! Fighting with our feelings and trying to push them away takes up a lot of energy and can get in the way of doing important things. Fighting or ignoring our feelings usually makes us feel worse in the end and keeps us struggling for longer; we may start to feel stuck, as if we just keep walking the same old road over and over again.

Urge surfing

The concept of urge surfing helps people to understand the skill of acceptance. We find it can be helpful to describe it in the following way, tailored to each individual's needs:

Surfers are really good at riding on top of waves. They do not stay on the beach to avoid the waves altogether, because that would not be surfing at all. However, they do not try to fight the waves by crashing through the middle of them. The surfers have learned to 'go with the waves'. We can learn to do the same. If we don't spend our time avoiding and fighting with emotions, they will naturally come and go. Sometimes they will be small, sometimes they will be really, really big. This can feel scary, but just like with surfing, we can still do it in exactly the same way. If we keep breathing, pay attention to our body and our emotions, we will notice that it will pass.

It can be helpful to show video clips of surfers riding large waves. There are online videos about urge surfing as an ACT skill and some of these can be suitable, particularly with your support to discuss the clips afterwards.

Passengers on the bus

The 'passengers on the bus' metaphor described earlier can also be used to explore the concept of acceptance. In the metaphor, the bus driver finds that they have a bus full of noisy, hostile (perhaps smelly) passengers shouting directions to them. The driver wishes the passengers were not there or would at least quit shouting.

The driver also learns that they can in fact drive the bus in any direction they want, even with the passengers shouting and posturing (indicating the possibility of values-based actions in the face of difficult thoughts and strong emotions). There are some excellent videos of this metaphor on popular video-streaming sites. In a group setting, this could be acted out, should there be a group of willing participants. This metaphor can be used to good effect with some people with milder learning disabilities, although our experience is that some people struggle with this metaphor and may require a different approach.

Tailoring metaphors

As discussed in Chapter 6, metaphors can be tailored to the person's interests. Take the example of a person with an interest in boxing. They may consider acceptance in terms of the willingness to move in towards an opponent, rather than follow the instinct to back away from the other person. For someone who has an interest in outdoor sports, you may talk about the idea of a tug-of-war versus dropping the rope. If their interest is computer games, you may talk about approaching the enemy rather than avoiding it.

Dropping the struggle

Ultimately, avoiding different activities, places, conversations (and the many other examples of avoidance) are really about the avoidance of uncomfortable bodily sensations resulting from difficult thoughts and emotions. Gentle and gradual exercises can be offered that help a person to notice and sit with bodily responses in different contexts. The physical experience of emotional pain or unwanted emotions will be unique to each individual so do check this out thoroughly during early sessions. Examples include a racing heart, rapid breathing, a heavy feeling in the chest, shaky hands, wobbly legs... (the list goes on). It is helpful to collaboratively identify the physical features of unwanted emotional experience for each individual.

Adopting different postures

It can be useful to invite the person to adopt different body postures and be curious about the different sensations they experience. They can try loosening their body around those sensations – not trying to rid themselves of the sensation, just dropping the fight against those sensations (which often shows up as tension in the body). Try to model and take part in the exercise along with the person so that they feel more comfortable doing it. Invite the person to breathe into whatever shape they have made their body into, to notice how it feels, and be curious about that body shape. Invite the person to notice how different body shapes feel different. Encourage the person to allow whatever feelings arise.

Difficulties with acceptance typically manifest in the body: we often hold our body in a tense way in an attempt to guard against our experiences. As an antidote, it is helpful to experiment with letting go of bodily tension as a means of allowing remaining bodily experiences to be whatever they will be.

To open up in the body, the following elements can be helpful:

- Invite the person to loosen their tongue in their mouth.
- Invite the person to gently move and loosen their jaw.
- Invite the person to gently allow their stomach to relax without holding it in. Most of us 'hold in' our stomachs most of the time without noticing.

Some people may not wish to try this if they feel self-conscious, but, for those who do, it can really help in reducing tension.

Alternatively, use a 'Chinese finger trap' (although it is not actually of Chinese origin). This is a paper tube; if you put a finger in at each end and try to pull them out, the tube tightens, and the fingers get stuck. This can be a fun way to demonstrate the struggle. This both amuses people and brings the concept to life. If you don't have a Chinese finger trap, you will need to carefully explain the exercise as many people will not have heard of them; or suggest/play one of the many YouTube videos showing them being used.

Another practical and effective exercise to explain the concept of 'dropping the struggle' can be to physically demonstrate 'dropping the mental tug of war'. This can be done in session using a piece of string, an actual rope or even a scarf. By holding the rope taut all day, constantly, a person's focus is always one hundred percent on the rope. This can be physically exhausting and doesn't allow us to pay attention to anything or anybody else around us. Literally dropping the rope (metaphorical version of the struggle) allows a person to free up their hands, body and mind. They can then choose to pivot towards something else that matters. They know that the rope (difficult thoughts/feelings) continues to exist yet choose to move towards a valued life direction despite its presence.

These kinds of exercises can also lead into drama or role-play-based techniques. Some people may enjoy acting as if they were a favourite famous person or character to see how that feels. It could also (with careful preparation and agreement) involve practising/role-playing emotionally challenging situations. Approaches can be tailored to the person in question, but examples include:

- sparking up a conversation with a new acquaintance
- saying no to another person's requests or demands
- going to a new place for the first time.

These allow the person to rehearse feeling some of the emotions associated with these challenging tasks. At the same time, they practise noticing the emotions, breathing into them, and carrying on with doing the important things anyway. Assertiveness exercises can be highly valuable here, because this is an area in which so many people we meet experience difficulty, even during role-plays. Of course, there are overlaps here with the 'doing' part of the toolkit, which focuses on values-oriented actions.

Taking up space

'Taking up space' exercises can be a follow-on or an alternative to the above exercises. When we feel anxious, guilty or sad, there can be tendency to hold this in our bodies: for example, physically contracting and tensing, dropping shoulders and stooping/curling. While this is at times a normal response, it can be helpful to practise expanding around difficult sensations and emotions. This can be done by raising the arms widely whilst breathing in, stretching and taking in as much space as possible. This can be done to the rhythm of calm breath cycles. Then try raising the hands up as high as possible.

Some people may initially feel self-conscious and reluctant. Of course, people should feel invited rather than obliged to engage in tasks. However, if suggestions for exercises are presented in a light-hearted or playful way (depending on what works for the particular person), many people may be willing to have a go. This is especially true if modelled by the therapist in the first instance and then completed alongside the person. If supporters are present, they would be expected to do the same.

This theme of 'taking up space' despite strong emotions can be built upon with subsequent exercises: for example, walking/striding confidently around a room or role-playing social situations whilst exhibiting a bold or positive posture, and observing how this feels compared to role-playing the same scenario with a shrinking or avoidant posture.

Should the individual be willing, they can lie on the floor in a 'star fish' shape, with arms, fingertips, legs and toes stretched out as much as possible and breathing in. It is difficult to be angry or hold on to difficult emotions in this position! Of course, consider any mobility issues prior to embarking on any of the tasks discussed here.

Compassion

Compassion is not explicitly named as one of the six evidence-based elements of the psychological flexibility model which underpins ACT. However, there is increasing evidence around the importance of compassion. Many clinicians interweave elements of compassion into ACT work due to the compatibility of these approaches (Tirch, Schoendorff & Silberstein, 2014). Many of the skills in each of the Hexaflex domains can be considered acts of self-compassion. Examples would be defusing and making room for thoughts and emotions linked to self-destructive patterns of behaviour, and holding lightly self-conceptualizations of being 'bad' or 'damaged' in some way. Also, many people hold personal values around kindness or helping others.

In terms of a technical definition, Gilbert and Choden (2013) defined compassion as 'a sensitivity to suffering in self and others with a commitment to try to alleviate and prevent it' (p.94). Building on this definition, Gilbert and colleagues have outlined three 'flows' of compassion: self-focused compassion, compassion towards others, and receptiveness to compassion from others.

Within the Feelings part of the toolkit, we most commonly incorporate self-compassion skills, since these arguably allow the most direct route to making room for strong emotions. However, being psychologically open to the compassion of others is very pertinent for many people experiencing psychological distress, as is the cultivation of a compassionate approach to others.

Accessible compassionate approaches

These exercises are likely to be suitable for people with a less significant learning disability, since they involve a degree of abstract thinking: imagining the advice of another or imagining a future self.

Older wise self

Invite the person to consider the advice that an older, even wiser, version of themselves would give to them about their current context and struggles. There are various ways to make this more accessible. The person can draw a picture of their imagined older self or just talk through things that they have experienced and worked through earlier in their lives.

To prompt discussion, it may also be helpful to search online for clips of older people giving advice to their younger selves. On a flipchart, the individual could draw an outline of a person to depict themselves in the future (or this could be more detailed and artistic, should they so wish!). Together with the therapist, they could say out loud or write down statements that the older version of themselves might say. The therapist can support the writing of these statements if that would be helpful for the individual. For each statement, one by one, walk up to the flipchart and stick them onto the body outline.

In our experience, this can be a powerful way of eliciting self-compassion with opportunities for discussion throughout the course of the activity. The therapist can note the individual's body language and facial expressions as they add each statement onto the body outline in order to gauge feelings around the task.

CASE STUDY: Samira

Samira was a middle-aged lady living with a complex history. She lived in supported living accommodation with two other people. When she was feeling well, Samira was able to engage in supported employment and enjoyed a good social life. However, she also struggled with periods of low mood, spending lots of time feeling understandably angry about her past trauma. Samira often blamed herself for not stopping past events.

Through the course of ACT therapy Samira found the various exercises helpful, particularly the 'older wise self' task. She liked to imagine her older self putting her arm around her, telling her that things were going to get better for her, and that she was not to blame for bad things that had happened. Samira remained angry about her life experiences but experienced less shame.

She liked to repeat the exercise regularly and augmented this by putting a heavy blanket over her shoulders and hugging herself tightly. After using the exercise, Samira's shoulders and jaw appeared less tense, and she was better able to concentrate on tasks she liked to complete around the home. It also helped her to build up motivation to venture out of the house during periods of low mood.

Advice to a best friend

Another approach is to invite the person to consider what advice they would give to a good friend who was struggling with difficulties similar to their own. The person may then be better placed to advise and soothe themselves. The therapist can help to make this exercise more concrete by discussing the friend to whom they are giving advice and supporting the person to build this imaginary conversation. They could ask the person where they would be meeting up with the friend, what they would be doing together, and possibly give some 'starter' suggestions as to the type of advice. Therapists can build on this by inviting the person to consider what kind of tone of voice they would use when being kind towards a friend, and to practise this using this tone of voice with themselves.

CASE STUDY: Anna

Anna, in her early twenties, had been taken into the care of social services when she was three years old. Anna was adopted before she started secondary school. Due to many difficult life experiences, including frequent placement moves and regularly starting new schools as a result, Anna had developed cognitive fusion with a negative self-narrative. This included an entrenched belief that she was 'not good enough', that she was inferior to others and would always fail, so therefore may not even bother to try. Anna was able to work this through in the form of a role-play alongside her therapist.

The therapist played the role of the friend to whom Anna would offer advice (whilst imagining that she may be able to offer the same kind and compassionate advice to herself in practice). Within the role-play, Anna chose to meet the friend at a local coffee house, where they sat in a cosy spot by the fire.

Although Anna initially found the hypothetical situation bizarre, she gradually settled into the task with the therapist's prompting and maintenance of character. Anna used a soft tone of voice to speak to her friend in a gentle, warm and friendly manner. She advised her to reach for the stars and to follow her dreams. Anna told the imaginary friend to 'Live in the moment and choose to move towards what truly matters every day!' Anna advised her friend to prioritize time for self-care and reminded her that she is more than enough, just as she was.

Compassionate other

It can be helpful to invite the person to imagine a compassionate figure. A compassionate other may be a famous person or fictional character whom the person admires. It is usually better to avoid family or friends. Actual relationships with loved ones can be complex, and imagining those people can bring mixed perspectives, mindful of the often ever-changing dynamic of personal relationships.

'Compassionate other' was used with Catherine, whose case was first discussed in Chapter 4.

CASE STUDY: Catherine (2)

Catherine was fanatical about musical theatre and especially loved the film *The Wizard of Oz*. For Catherine, the key film character of Glinda the Good Witch, a fairy godmother-like character, encapsulated everything she would wish for from the figure of the compassionate other. The character was kind, friendly, gentle and caring. Within sessions, Catherine and the therapist would often consider the question 'And what might Glinda say about this?' For example, when Catherine expressed that she was 'not good enough' – 'I just can't do it; there is no point anymore; I fail every time I try' – Catherine was able to tap into her compassionate other figure, who would offer kind and calming words such as 'Take a deep breath and check in; drop anchor. These thoughts will pass: you are good enough and you have the strength to try again. You are strong and resilient.'

Repeated practice of this approach supported Catherine to move towards more regular self-compassion and slowly distance herself from her automatic habit of self-criticism.

Receiving compassion from others

Being able to receive compassion from others is an important part of psychological wellbeing. A person who is able to receive the compassion of others will be more likely to feel soothed and supported by helpful and caring people around them. They will also likely internalize this self-compassion over time and be better able to soothe themselves.

Acceptance skills are interlinked with this ability as well, since what is required is an ability to make room for the uncomfortable sensations that may arise for some people when receiving compassion from others. Practitioners can work with the person to notice their own responses when another person demonstrates acts of care towards them. Acceptance can be developed by noticing feelings and 'breathing into' parts of the body where sensations are arising.

This is a great skill that lends itself well to supporter involvement – there are ways that supporters may foster opportunities to practise this skill with the individual. The practitioner can offer opportunities for the supporter(s) or whole staff teams to discuss responses and consider ways to work through any difficulties that may arise when individuals may find it difficult to accept compassion from others.

It can be modelled between members of supporter teams too. For example, family or team members can offer each other compassion on a regular basis and in an open and transparent way in order for the person with intellectual disabilities to see this in action, and for this to become the 'norm'.

Being compassionate to others

Acts of compassion can be beneficial for the person and, of course, the recipient of that compassion. Being compassionate towards others can give a sense of satisfaction as well as improving relationships with others. Having a compassionate outlook more broadly is likely to mean that the person will in turn be more compassionate towards themselves over time.

Examples of compassionate approaches to others:

* Acts of kindness: one way that people can be compassionate towards

others is to engage in acts of kindness. There are many, many ways that this can be done, for example:

- offering to make a cup of tea for a friend, carer or supporter
- saying 'good morning' to people
- letting somebody in front of you at the till at the supermarket when they have fewer items than you do
- sending a hand-written note with a positive message to a friend, relative or supporter.

- Becoming involved in community activities that involve helping others, animals or the local area. This could come under values for lots of people but deserves a mention here as well. A person who is able to feel comforted and supported is likely to be somewhat buffered from ongoing psychological suffering.

  This is much like the case of Melanie discussed in Chapter 5. Identification of her love of animals and dogs in particular led her towards activities that she really valued, supporting her to engage in meaningful activities which truly mattered to her, and in turn having a positive impact on her overall physical health and management of health conditions such as diabetes (through increased exercise as a result of partaking in valued activities, rather than simply going to a gym).

- Complimenting someone – this may include thanking a family member for something they did that was appreciated, thanking a member of staff in a shop, sending a text message to a friend to let them know that you are grateful to have them in your life, or sending positive feedback after a positive customer service interaction.

- Donating items to a charity shop, or local cause. This could include creating a 'care package' of specific items much needed by charities such as helping those that are homeless, or helping individuals in crisis.

- Signing up to do voluntary work in the local community.

Challenges to compassion

Whilst compassion skills can be very helpful, it is to be expected that barriers and challenges will often emerge when a person begins to develop their compassion skills. One of the core yearnings described by Hayes (2019) relates to the longing for cohesion – humans tend to have a need to understand themselves and the world around them. Some people struggling with psychological distress may have experienced criticism and negative views of themselves. As discussed, people with intellectual disabilities are more disposed to this than most. This can mean that people may find self-compassion uncomfortable or confusing if they have internalized a view of themselves as being unworthy or in some way defective. Sometimes, it can feel easier to stick with negative self-concepts than to accept the initial discomfort of developing a more compassionate view.

People who have had difficult experiences at the hands of others may be in a state of vigilance to threat. They may initially equate being compassionate to themselves with weakness and thus vulnerability. More relaxed states can be feared due to a sense that it is only a matter of time before something bad happens again (Gilbert & Choden, 2013).

These challenges can often be managed by giving control to the person around pace and choice of activities, as well as modelling a sense of curiosity about whatever feelings come up. Acceptance skills can really help people to make room for whatever emotions arise. The wide range of literature in the field on compassion-focused therapy can provide further suggestions in respect to fears, blocks and resistance to compassion.

SUMMARY

+ Feeling skills are a key element of the Noticing, Feeling, Doing toolkit.

+ Acceptance skills are about making room for difficult feelings rather than engaging in excessive experiential avoidance. From a position of moving towards acceptance, a person becomes skilled in noticing the struggle as it arises and choosing to drop the struggle in order to free themselves up to take steps towards valued aspects of life.

+ Compassion-based approaches are another form of feeling skill and involve helping the person to nurture compassion towards themselves and others as well as being able to receive compassion from others.

+ People often struggle with feeling skills for understandable reasons. Using creative approaches and validating reactions can be helpful, as can linking the skills and valued actions to help build motivation.

See Appendix 2 for a summary of the Hexaflex in relation to feeling skills (as well as for noticing and doing skills).

Chapter 8

DOING SKILLS

The 'doing' skills outlined in this chapter relate to the 'Committed Action' aspects of the ACT Hexaflex, which are focused upon putting values into everyday action. This chapter outlines principles of planning: for example, setting reminders, making a timetable, overcoming internal and external barriers to completing activities, as well as grading of activities towards particular goals (considering one step at a time).

Committed Action

In many ways, there is little complexity with regard to the *concept* of Committed Action, at least providing that the concept of Values has been considered and established in a meaningful way. Committed Action is sometimes described as the part 'where the rubber hits the road' (in keeping with our roadmap analogy). Having identified what and who is important to them, we support the person to take specific actions that are consistent with those values. In Choice Point terms, these would be considered 'towards moves'.

For example, a person who values self-development/personal growth may begin to learn some new skills, such culinary or literacy skills, or may start a photography class. Someone else who values being kind to other people might plan how to do kind things for people they know, or consider how to resist acting in a grumpy or cross way to friends or family when they are feeling tired or overwhelmed. Committed Action would typically take the form of *observable behaviours*, such as by taking time out to go for a walk.

Evaluating Committed Action skills:

According to Wilson (2009), someone with well-developed committed-action skills will:

- work towards and do the things that matter to them, even in the face of disappointment or frustrating outcomes
- choose short-term and long-term goals that fit with what matters to them
- notice when they are doing things or have done things that don't fit with what matters to them, and can gently get back to doing more things that are important to them (i.e. get on the road again if they swerve off course, or take an unanticipated diversion)
- are not defensive when others, or they, notice that they are acting in ways that are inconsistent with their values.

Someone with less-developed Committed Action skills will likely:

- be driven by attempts to relieve difficult thoughts or feelings, which could be through inaction, avoidance, impulsiveness or persisting with unhelpful approaches
- talk often about what they must/mustn't do or should/shouldn't do
- have difficulty generating goals that are consistent with their values
- not seem to notice when their behaviour does not fit with their values or becomes fixated on their failure to maintain commitment to their goals.

Accessible approaches to establishing Committed Action

Once you have established a person's values, the next step is in translating these into committed actions – that is to say, specific goals that are consistent with personal values. Committed Action could refer to an almost infinite number of behaviours. The challenge is working with the person to identify possible values-based actions for them. People are often asked about their goals and sometimes struggle to identify them. On the face of it, this might seem a little like a lack of focus, drive or motivation. As we said in Chapter 4, in some services, such factors as these can even be an exclusion criterion for therapy. As intellectual disability practitioners we do not adopt this approach. Part of the process of therapy for many people is learning who they are and what matters to them. This is very much part of the therapy itself. Although we will ask people about their goals at the start of therapy, being unable to answer this question is not a significant issue. Even if a person is able to provide answers, we revisit this throughout the therapy in different ways as the process itself may lead to changes.

The use of visual materials, as ever, can be very useful in the domain of Committed Action. It can be useful to use or construct a list of possible day-to-day activities such as housekeeping, leisure and self-care, as well as activities that help others or contribute to the community. Visual materials are beneficial when people will struggle to think through how values may be shaped into specific activity-based goals.

Link the suggested activities to the values identified; otherwise, you will simply have a list of likes and dislikes that may or may not give an accurate picture. The practitioner can also use their own knowledge or initiative to determine which actions or activities may be values-congruent, rather than relying on the person to be able to think of some.

For example, a person may establish that being kind is an important value, or perhaps you as a practitioner have tentatively deduced this value from the issues that upset them. The person frequently becomes upset when others are bullied/teased or when they themselves have not behaved in a kind way. If you have agreed together that this person values kindness, you may need to establish the kind actions they wish to engage in. We recommend offering some concrete options where necessary as some people may still find this difficult from a cognitive perspective.

Alternatively, you could generate a list of kind actions and then present the person with the accessible Easy-Read Bullseye diagram (Figure 5.1). Invite the person to pick which actions they currently do, and which they would like to do more of in each domain (e.g. friends/family). The kind actions generated might be:

- make a coffee for someone
- buy myself something nice
- have a nice bath
- thank someone for their help.

You may then consider different areas of life such as:

- family
- friends
- work
- leisure.

From this, you may identify that the person is already doing plenty of kind actions with family but not in work. Alternatively, you may note that the person isn't doing any kind actions in any domain despite this being an important value. In this way, you are working together to shape up a person's values-based goals.

We sometimes use an adapted version of the Russ Harris 'Willingness and Action Plan', which can be helpful in breaking down goals into more manageable steps and identifying potential barriers. This is in effect a summary of the values-based goals, complete with potential barriers and ways to overcome them. This can be difficult for some people to do without support. It may involve some guidance from the practitioner if they have relevant knowledge of the person and their wider system. If not, you could invite input from supporters, provided this does not involve the supporter confusing their own views with that of the people they are supporting.

You can download the adapted Willingness and Action Plan worksheet at https://digitalhub.jkp.com/redeem (or scan the QR code) using the voucher code UAHJYLC.

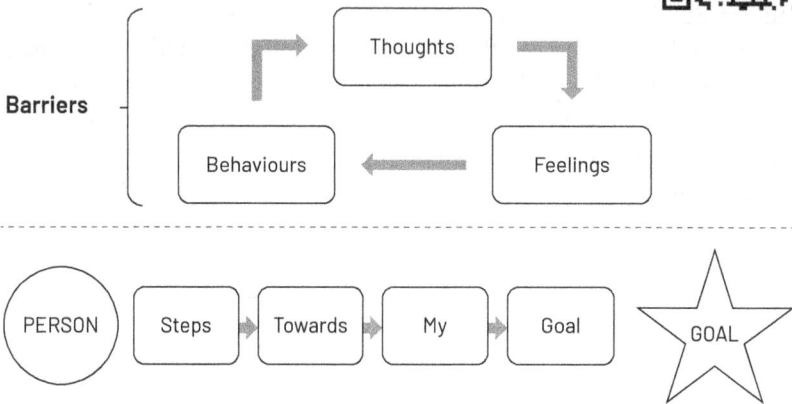

Figure 8.1 *Lifeline exercise*

We have found that the use of physicalizing exercises can be an excellent way to assist people to identify goals and the committed actions needed to achieve them. The 'lifeline' exercise (Figure 8.1) involves assisting the person to map out their goals, identify steps towards them and recognize what their current position may be. It can also be helpful to map out alongside noting the associated thoughts, feelings and behaviours. Once these areas are identified, these may be mapped on to pieces of paper that can be placed on the floor in a manner similar to Figure 8.1. The person is encouraged to walk along various paths, including towards their goal, looking back when the goal has been achieved. They experience what it is like to reach their goals, to be stuck in a thoughts/behaviours/feelings cycle, or to make the first step. As well as motivating people into Committed Action, this exercise can also be said to help with Defusion and Self-as-Context.

Other Committed Action ('doing skills') exercises can include the 'epitaph' exercise – 'What do you want people to say about you at your funeral?' For people who may find thinking about their death as either too abstract or distressing you can ask 'What do you want people to say about you at your 80th birthday party?' This has the bonus of simultaneously offering a message of hope about living a long and healthy life.

It is also important to explore the origin of any identified personal goals.

CASE STUDY

One of us (ST) worked with a person who struggled with OCD focused on germs. The person had been saying for many years that he would like to work at a recycling plant. Given the obvious conflict with the person's presenting difficulties and the goal, this merited further exploration.

It transpired that this goal was one that the person had in fact had since childhood. Under pressure from his family to have 'normal' future goals, and in the absence of a clear sense of his own identity, he continued to express a wish to do this job, without fully recognizing the barriers inherent in this type of work.

Using ACT-based activities to explore goals should minimize the chances of misunderstanding the person and will help them to explore their own life goals. This process can take time as the person (hopefully) gains more insight into themselves.

How to engage in Committed Action

Behavioural activation approaches

Behavioural activation is a recommended approach to the treatment of depression (Jahoda et al., 2017; NICE, 2022). With the support of their practitioner, people feel pleasure and achievement being given activities structured into their day with the goal of encouraging engagement in them despite their mood at that point. This shifts an emphasis (that is present for some people) from waiting until they feel better to engage in more activity, to building activity patterns that, when established, lead to greater life satisfaction. Developing graded activity schedules based on value-based activities can be a powerful way to utilize ACT principles. These can be adjusted according to the person's needs and delivered in a step-by-step manner.

In terms of increasing the accessibility of behavioural activation approaches, many people with intellectual disabilities will use visual planners, whether pictorial or written. However, some people we have worked with have not been fully involved in developing their planners. It may not be that the timetable represents what matters to them.

The person could be supported to develop more specific weekly plans where the person adds the values-based goals/activities that they have identified as meaningful. Where necessary, they could be encouraged by support staff to consider these elements when developing their planners. Visuals can be used to represent hierarchies (e.g. a ladder, where the practitioner can highlight the possibility of 'going down a few rungs' where momentum is not maintained). Alternative analogies can be used dependent on individual interest and preferences. For example, in the case of Catherine, a long and winding Yellow Brick Road contains twists and turns that may lead a person away from the 'pot of gold' (values) at the end, noting that a person always has a choice to move towards the things that matter. Inclusion of such strategies may enhance the likelihood of people regularly attending their appointments.

CASE STUDY: Melanie (2)

An example of the importance of values-based behavioural activation can be seen in the case of Melanie (as described in Chapter 5). Her visual planner included activities such as trips to the gym. Exercise was something that staff felt she *should* be doing because of her physical health status, diabetes and obesity. Melanie had no desire whatsoever to do this, nor to reduce her intake of biscuits alongside her hot drink at multiple times throughout the day. By engaging Melanie in values work in a meaningful way, her staff support team were able to tailor her activity schedule towards the things that truly mattered to her. Through her voluntary roles within the community and the local animal shelter, she became more active, her mood improved, and she lost weight as a by-product. This highlights the need to think in creative ways and outside of the box when possible.

Ensure that individual planners are developed in line with individual communication and literacy skills. One of the authors has witnessed in the past that a person's schedule had been written using words when a person is unable to read. Similarly, specific times had been written on the planner using numbers, but the individual was unable to tell the time using the clocks that he had available to him. It is vital to check out a person's abilities from the outset in order to flexibly tailor unique individual plans.

Enlisting support

Once values-based goals and the relevant steps to move towards these have been identified, a key difference or adaptation here is this that support may be needed to actualize the goals.

Note that it is not only people with intellectual disabilities who can struggle with change. Supporters may also need to adjust to supporting in new ways. It is the responsibility of the practitioner to help them to do so. It is therefore important to have a clearly defined contract, written or verbal, which covers the expectations and responsibilities of both the person and their supporter. Involvement of supporters, where appropriate, in discussion around the identified committed actions and the values behind them may help the supporter to appreciate their importance in helping people live values-based lives.

For example, we have worked with people who wish to have more independence from their supporters. This can require new care- and risk-management plans and discussions with supporters to ensure they understand the person's wishes and are engaged with supporting them. We have also worked with people who wish to attend particular activities but have found the activities curtailed due to staff shifts. These types of systemic factors will need to be explored to avoid setting the person up to fail.

To once again consider Melanie, her staff team gave comments during the end of an intervention feedback session. This was a collaborative meeting alongside Melanie, the therapist and her staff team. They commented that they had had no idea exercise and keeping fit was not a value of hers in any way. An assumption had been made based on the status of her physical health. Through meaningful engagement and realization of a person's values – the things that truly matter to them – positive changes can ensue.

Exposure

For someone working on anxiety difficulties, exposure work may include a stepwise hierarchy of actions related to a specific fear (i.e. graded exposure). When using ACT, the goals are values-driven. Therefore, exposure aims to achieve a values-based goal, even when difficult thoughts and feelings show up, rather than simply aiming to extinguish the anxiety.

Within ACT based exposure work, the emphasis is not on the *reduction* in anxiety. Rather, the aim is to shift the agenda of the person from avoidance of negative emotions to increasing flexible behaviour according to what matters to the person. Russ Harris describes exposure as 'moving with the TIMES' – exposure that flexibly exposes the person to thoughts, images, memories, emotions and sensations.

It is often difficult to achieve this where a person's agenda remains even partially tied to 'feeling better' or the removal of specific aversive experiences. It is up to the practitioner to judge how much emphasis to put on this distinction. However, it is generally helpful to encourage mindfully experiencing emotions as they arise and subside, rather than having an agenda of reduction or elimination of aversive experiences.

Practice

The importance of practice may need to be emphasized. Some people tend to try something once and conclude it does not work.

We sometimes compare doing something new to trying to learn a musical instrument. We would not expect to pick up a guitar and immediately start playing complex tunes; we know that we will need to practise to improve. In the same way, encourage the person to practise the skills they are learning in order to develop confidence and a sense of self-efficacy. We would recommend that supporters are involved. Through practice, eventually some ways of behaving may become more second nature. The ACT model places the concept of 'doing things differently' at the heart of the therapy. Therefore, practice is key.

Practice can also occur within sessions. We would encourage this experiential element as much as possible. Some people will also need support building their practices into a daily routine. Lapses of practice should, of course, be normalized, but at the same time the practitioner can provide encouragement. They can help with problem-solving around how to increase home practice and skills use within day-to-day life. We have all had experience of the challenge of behaving and relating in new ways, and the ease in which we can slip back into old habits.

Barriers and solutions

We have encountered a range of barriers when supporting people to do more of what matters in their lives, and consequently with experience we have developed potential removers of such 'roadblocks'.

Roadblock 1: Memory

Difficulties with recall from therapy sessions is common. Some people struggle to recall material without specific cues. If this is the case, they will equally struggle to use material when needed.

When people can recall limited amounts from a session, this can also suggest that the material was delivered in too complex a way or in the wrong format in the first place. It is not always a difficulty with recall, but rather with attention, comprehension and storage of the experience.

Removing the roadblock
It is possible to facilitate recall through the support of others (family/carer/paid staff involvement) and co-production of creative reminders about actions, such as:

- *Reminder alarms or use of apps on mobile phone*: Are there particular times during a typical week when the individual finds it particularly difficult to make a choice that moves them towards valued aspects of life? Through collaborative consideration between the individual, the practitioner and the support network, prompts may be developed to serve as a reminder around the time when difficulties arise.

- *Posters/creative notes placed in convenient locations*: For example, if the kitchen is a trigger area for making decisions that may not align with values, reminder notes could be placed on the cupboard door to encourage a check-in regarding decision-making and a pause to consider next steps. Posters/notes may be developed by the individual, perhaps using felt-tips /paper and pen or using a computer package. The aim of this task is both to serve as a reminder and to encourage a shared approach between individuals and their support network to work towards an agreed aim.

- *Making it a mission/provision of a 'role' for undertaking actions*: For example, if the role is photography, making a choice to take photographs of valued aspects of life, and making it a mission to do so. (This is closely linked to the Catching What Matters approach discussed in Chapter 5.) Can this mission be shared and encouraged by supporters?

CASE STUDY: Mobile phone app as prompt

One of the authors worked with a person who froze/dissociated in the mornings when getting up and ready for the day, particularly when tired or when anticipating a stressful event. It would not have been possible to engage in discussions with her at this point, but in therapy sessions we identified that doing a grounding exercise soon after getting up would be an appropriate and helpful 'towards move'. She disliked supporters' guidance and prompts at this difficult time. She was adept with technology and the use of her phone, so we used apps to prompt her with using her grounding techniques. This assisted with utilization of skills at a time when it would be difficult to recall, without needing the involvement of others.

Roadblock 2: Motivation

Where a person describes difficulties with motivation, we need to identify what might underlie it. It might be anxiety, learned helplessness (a sense of lack of control as a result of repeated negative experiences), low self-esteem or a lack of available support. However, some people may say that they 'couldn't be bothered', or 'didn't have time', or indicate a lack of motivation through their non-verbal or verbal behaviour. It never truly means 'cannot be bothered', since we all, deep down, wish for meaningful and satisfying lives.

Removing the roadblock

If people seem to lack motivation to achieve their goals and make positive steps forwards, we suggest that you may not yet have captured together what truly matters to the person. If it matters, then by definition the person should feel motivated to move towards it.

In this circumstance, revisiting values may be needed. If you feel confident that the values and goals are correct, we suggest you explore the factors that can underlie an apparent lack of motivation and consider ways to overcome those barriers. For example, anxiety may be overcome by returning to creative hopelessness, Defusion and physicality exercises (such as the lifeline exercise). Low self-esteem and learned helplessness can be addressed by focusing on some easy-to-achieve early gains or some prior work on self-esteem.

Roadblock 3: Resistance or views of others

In our experience, this is a common roadblock. Whilst the person may be motivated and excited to move towards new areas of life, most people with intellectual disabilities rely on others to help them in their daily lives. Most supporters are doing their best (and there are many great supporters), but some may not have the right mentoring or training to provide the necessary support. Supporters may naturally hold differing values about the things they feel the person should be doing. How this is managed by supporters and practitioners will be important. Without well-tailored day-to-day support, the person may feel disempowered and not continue their efforts.

Equally, it may be that an outcome of therapy is that the person decides that what they want from therapy may be different from the original goal suggested either by them or their supporter. For example, others may have wanted the person to engage more in their day service activity. Yet, through exploration and increased sense of self, they may leave therapy with a clearer alternative view on what they want for their future, which may be something completely different to initial plans.

CASE STUDY: Lee

One of us worked with Lee, who came to his initial therapy session with his partner Tom. Tom had clear views on what he wanted Lee to achieve in sessions. He wanted Lee to do more around the house and to stop arguments. This point of view was enhanced by Lee's family, who described Lee as lazy and difficult. Over time, and through exploration of their values and emotions in the therapeutic space away from his husband, Lee became more aware of dissatisfaction with their marriage and decided to seek a divorce. Therapy outcomes are not always well received by supporters but can in fact be an indicator that therapy has been useful to the person.

As practitioners, we should certainly seek to work effectively with supporters. At the same time, we may need to withstand some counter-opinions from others in the person's life when the person has been able to communicate what matters to them.

Removing the roadblock

If you are encountering resistance or opposing views from supporters, some work may need to be at a systemic level, providing the person consents. It may be that the supporters simply do not understand the role of therapy and are certainly unlikely to understand ACT. What may appear to be resistance needs to be explored and understood as a valid perspective.

At a more extreme level, if you were concerned that the supporter was being abusive, a referral to social services may need to be made in respect of issues with the support the person receives. Sometimes what can appear to be over-involvement or being controlling may be a symptom of something more severe. Referrals to professionals such as social workers may help if the supporters are failing to help the person to achieve their goals, or if an increase or change in the type of support is required. The involvement of an advocate may also be helpful. Sometimes, the apparent resistance of others may be due to a lack of shared understanding of the issues among all relevant stakeholders.

It is not unusual for multiple perspectives to be evident within the vast networks that can be involved in someone's life. In this case, collaboratively developing a formulation with not only the person but also the supporters may help to shift attributions and help the person to feel more supported.

CASE STUDY: Greta

Greta lived with her late mother's friend Rose. Rose was an older lady (Greta now referred to her as Mum) whose husband and son had both died suddenly in a car crash. Floundering following her bereavement, she began unconsciously relying on Greta for her emotion needs.

Greta was going to a day service she disliked and felt unable to do activities away from Rose, as she felt guilty when doing so. She expressed a wish to get a boyfriend, have a family like her siblings had, and focus on hobbies such as baking. However, she was blocked at every turn. Rose stated that there was little point in Greta doing hobbies because she 'never liked anything she did' and reportedly said that finding a boyfriend would never work. In therapy, Greta sadly told the therapist there was no point in even trying because things would never change, and that she had no choice but to continue the life she was living. She sobbed in every session

The practitioner worked with Greta and her supporters to try to encourage them to think in a more flexible way about Greta's wishes. Greta was referred to an advocate to try to support her in creating a life that mattered, but the 'learned helplessness' was startling.

In Chapter 10 we discuss how to work with the wider system from an ACT perspective, as it was clear that working directly with Greta would be ineffective without concurrent shifts in the system.

Roadblock 4: Thoughts and feelings get in the way

Fusion with thoughts and feelings can be a barrier to living a full, valued life. It is highly likely that when people start making new 'towards moves', they will experience an increase in difficult thoughts and feelings. At this point, Defusion and acceptance skills will be extremely important. For someone with an intellectual disability, taking control and making changes may be scary. It may even seem impossible. As we have said, some people can struggle significantly with Defusion, most likely due to their neurological differences. This means that they cannot easily think at a 'meta' level (i.e. thinking about thinking). From their point of view, if it feels bad, then it is bad.

Impulsivity is a common difficulty. Many people with intellectual disabilities have issues with executive functioning, and some have ADHD. A person with these challenges may have difficulty in identifying their thoughts and feelings before acting.

Removing the roadblock

Focused work on Defusion (Chapter 6) can be helpful if this seems to be in the person's zone of proximal development (in other words, if this skill appears to be something they could be expected to develop with support). Where possible, it can be helpful to identify the specific thoughts. Examples would be thoughts about not being good enough, thoughts that they will not be able to do something, or thoughts about the therapeutic process (or the therapist).

Acceptance skills can be helpful in terms of making room for anxiety and any other emotions that may arise. Naming the emotion and/or where it shows up in the body can help, as can talking about 'bringing the emotion along for the ride'. Examples of difficult things the person has done in the past (and overcome) can be helpful. This could include coming along to the therapy sessions for the first time. Support may also be needed: perhaps it is simply too challenging to do something new in the face of difficult thoughts and feelings without assistance.

Finally, it may be necessary to return to creative hopelessness should the person still be focused upon an agenda of emotional control and/or experiential avoidance. Revisiting the Choice Point and reminding about values may aid motivation.

Roadblock 5: Availability of options

Many people with intellectual disabilities continue to experience narrower lives than others, although this could arguably be considered to be changing. Through therapy you may collaboratively establish that more presence at social groups is an important goal. However, this may be considered impossible due to staff shifts or transport issues: access to activities that are offered at the appropriate level may be limited; and insufficient staff support may also reduce people's options.

Removing the roadblock

Following discussion and agreement with the person, we sometimes engage in exploratory work around available services and make referrals for the appropriate support. Often, there are in fact a variety of possible services that people can access, but they may not be widely known about. We have also found it useful for local intellectual disability services to map relevant services for people. It is useful for the practitioner to have a good awareness of what is available locally and to alert the person and their supporters to what exists.

CASE STUDY: Sally

Sally had been working with a practitioner for some time. Through ACT-based approaches, she had decided she would like to work with animals. When this was raised with the third sector organization supporting Sally, the practitioner was told that Sally could not do so because she had an intellectual disability and therefore was not covered by insurance.

There were no risk issues towards animals. Sally was a kind and gentle woman. The organization was advised that this was discriminatory and that it should be challenged. Her social worker was alerted. With support to the employer the issue was resolved, and Sally was able to begin to explore available options. Sally eventually got a part-time job in an animal sanctuary.

Sadly, society still discriminates in a whole variety of ways, and this is what some people face. We must be alert to the stigma, discrimination and lack of understanding that still exists. Part of our work may be in challenging such situations.

People may have person-centred plans or support plans developed by third-sector agencies or social workers. It will be important to ensure any work you do with someone sits alongside or supports such work. Practitioners may be able to be involved in annual support package reviews. If so, they can support the incorporation of ACT approaches and person-centred, values-based goals within such interventions. Where a CCaRM formulation (see Chapter 2) may have been collaboratively developed by individuals and support teams, this can be a helpful anchor for reviews of progress and a tool to identify areas where further support/input may be helpful.

SUMMARY

* Doing skills are possibly the most important and in some ways the simplest to understand. They are the actions that transform a person's life.

* That said, there are various potential barriers ('roadblocks'), both in the wider system and for individuals that need to be overcome to make meaningful change, which are not always so simple but require practitioners to problem solve.

* Often people with ID have little control over their lives, and as such, many of the roadblocks must be addressed with supporters and involved professionals.

See Appendix 2 for a summary of the Hexaflex in relation to doing skills (as well as for noticing and feeling skills).

Chapter 9

SELF-REFLECTION

The willingness and ability to engage in reflective practice is an important element of being an ACT practitioner. Noticing our own responses and increasing self-awareness can improve practitioner skills and enrich the therapeutic relationship. Meaningful implementation of ACT principles within our own lives can increase wellbeing and help develop a greater appreciation of the benefits and challenges of living according to values in day-to-day life. As ACT practitioners, we should, of course, aim to practise what we preach, with all the inevitable human fallibility and challenges that this entails. This chapter covers ways in which this can be worked towards. It discusses the role of supervision and how to use existing models of reflective practice in an ACT-informed way, which will impact not only on our clinical work but also on our ability to self-reflect.

Being present

Wilson (2009) highlights the importance of practitioners being in the present moment during the course of their practice in order to truly listen to and be present with people. Of course, we are human and will be influenced by what has happened from one day to the next. However, during a session with an individual, we should strive to remain as present and mindful as we can, making this our aim. If we ourselves are emotionally avoidant, defensive, become fused with our thoughts, or are not present due to poor mindfulness skills, this will impact upon our clinical work.

A practitioner who lacks confidence may find themselves unable to sit with a person's suffering due to the way in which this triggers the practitioner's feelings and thoughts of inadequacy. This could inadvertently reinforce the person's emotional avoidance and fusion with negative thoughts.

A practitioner who has poor attention skills and a tendency to daydream and does not seek to improve this via regular mindfulness practice may periodically not hear people at vital moments. Some people with intellectual disabilities may be less likely to notice, assert themselves or act upon it when this occurs, but this does not make it any less important to address. Practitioners may find themselves moving between two states: clear focus in the unfolding interaction and distractedness to other matters. This is especially true when they face the dual challenge of balancing many spinning plates in their clinical role and busy personal lives.

Continually monitoring one's own focus and returning to the present moment is like exercising a muscle. Over time it leads to greater present-moment skills. Being fully present, aware of both the nuances of the therapeutic interaction and the ways in which this may change and evolve from session to session, enhances one's ability to truly reflect. This is particularly relevant during clinical supervision about the therapeutic process, an individual's progress or potential barriers to engagement throughout the course of the work. An example can be seen in Catherine's case.

CASE STUDY: Catherine (3)

Through completion of session rating scales (as described previously), Catherine was able to ask the therapist to allow her more time to speak by rating the therapist's 'listening skills' as 5 out of 10.

By letting the therapist know, Catherine was able to open up a conversation about her needs. The therapist endeavoured to offer plenty of time for her to talk about the things on her mind. Catherine was able to open up about a previous difficult relationship. Together, they were able to consider the ways in which this influenced her current presentation and patterns of interaction. The therapist had also discussed this case in supervision; there always seemed to be a sense that Catherine had more to her story than she initially disclosed. This was hidden behind a chatty and talkative demeanour, smiling often and putting the needs of others first.

Through reflection and open, professionally honest and transparent discussion, a shift in the therapeutic dynamic was possible.

Reflective practice
What is reflective practice?

Self-awareness can also be enhanced by regular reflective practice about our own thought patterns and tendencies. Reflective practice can be defined as 'learning through and from experience towards gaining new insights of self and practice' (Finlay, 2008, p.1). It involves the willingness to look inwards, without defence, at one's own practice, at one's own ways of relating and how one's own thoughts, feelings, behaviours, past experiences and current view of the world impacts upon the other(s) and vice versa.

Reflective practice can take place in a myriad of ways. It should form an integral part of practice and can occur at any moment. It may also take the form of structured reflective practice sessions, or reflective space within supervision. Where possible, we would also recommend recording sessions to reflect upon afterwards, although this requires ethical consideration.

Some people find it useful to keep a reflective diary. Reflection can be at an individual or group level. The way in which reflective practice takes place depends upon whatever works best for the practitioner. What is vital is that it occurs in some form.

Themes for reflection
Power
We have already discussed the influence of power in our work. As practitioners, we can sometimes fail to appreciate what it may feel like for the person or their supporters to meet with someone they view as a professional or expert. We may not view ourselves as being in a position of power.

We can only truly reflect upon the person/supporter experience if we have truly listened to and spent time with the person in an open and vulnerable way. One way to ensure reflection includes the influence of power and privilege may be to use the Power Threat Meaning framework (Chapter 2). We recommend keeping the theme of power 'on the menu' when engaging in reflective work.

Our own use of ACT
Practitioners should reflect upon their modelling of the use of ACT principles during their work. Are we expecting more from the person than we would of ourselves? Do we truly appreciate what it is like to engage in ACT work? Do we buy in to the model on a day-to-day basis?

A practitioner should utilize ACT if it fits with their core values. In Choice Point terms, the use of ACT must be a 'towards move' in the service of values-based goals. We do not recommend using ACT if you do not believe in and apply ACT principles in your own life, which can include a true appreciation of the challenges in maintaining regular present moment, acceptance, Defusion or other ACT exercises.

A true appreciation of and engagement with ACT in our own lives enables us to model its use to others. In doing so, we do not mean modelling a 'perfect' response. We are referring to a genuine offering of the realities of using ACT in everyday life. This can include the positive impact but also the challenges, stumbling blocks and frustrations. We may name occasions where we have become fused with particular thoughts or rules, or we may describe difficulties raising particular topics from feelings of anxiety.

The use of ACT can also be implicit, just monitoring our own moment-by-moment experiences during sessions and reflecting upon and making use of what we notice. We may decide to name the internal processes that are occurring: this will model both noticing and naming. At the same time, we may be describing a transference reaction or a mirroring process that, by naming it, opens up new and important conversations. For example, we may find that we feel irritated by or even angry with someone, or with their situation. Being able to notice and name and reflect upon this in the moment may give the person permission to own the emotion for themselves.

By engaging in the use of ACT ourselves, and modelling this in all its facets, we show our common humanity and help to ameliorate the influence of power. When we avoid presenting ourselves as experts, but rather as flawed human beings with common struggles, we show to others, who may initially view us in an expert role, that we are all indeed 'in the same boat.' We are putting our money where our mouths are!

While we may not have all the answers, we do possess a valuable toolkit of skills that can support others (and ourselves) in navigating their own lives. Alongside this, we are committed to meeting people where they are at, while also staying true to where we are at, fostering a genuine, open and honest relationship.

Personal disclosure

The use of disclosure should be used judiciously and must be formulation-driven. This is an area we find is a common theme in reflective spaces, hence it is highlighted here. Whereas in some therapeutic models (such as the psychodynamic tradition) self-disclosure is not used at all, this is acceptable when using the ACT model, provided it is considered useful for the person.

Different practitioners will have different views on how much disclosure is acceptable. When working with people with intellectual disabilities some caution has to be present. Some people coming to therapy will have a lack of understanding of appropriate and inappropriate conversation and can appear unboundaried. Some people will also have little understanding of therapy boundaries. In such cases, less disclosure may be advised. The philosophy 'we are all in the same boat' does not mean that we disclose vast amounts of personal information: we still consider what is *therapeutically useful* to share. Usually, this can be done with very little disclosure of personal details, since it is more about personal responses. For example, a practitioner may share that they struggle with thoughts about being good enough at certain things.

It is probably not necessary to go into past events that may have shaped and reinforced the occurrence of these thoughts or beliefs. What it does mean is that we are prepared to make ourselves vulnerable by sharing some of ourselves when therapeutically helpful. Deciding when to do so may require space for reflection.

Your own Hexaflex

It can be useful spending time considering ourselves as practitioners in relation to the Hexaflex domains at regular intervals. This will increase self-awareness and enables us to consider how we are connecting with others. It can be useful to do this in a general sense to understand our own ACT formulations and how this may impact our work. It can also be useful with respect to specific sessions or situations.

Take a specific conversation from a session and consider this in relation to the Hexaflex domains. We may reflect upon a conversation and realize that in that session we were more aligned with our own values than that of the person. We may also notice some thoughts that come up for us during the session from which we need to defuse. For example, a person describing their lack of progress may lead to strong thoughts that 'I'm not a good therapist'. This may be a pervasive narrative from which you need to defuse, or it could be a thought that is elicited in a specific situation, upon which you may need to reflect.

You might be someone who experiences unhelpful thoughts around their own competence or begins to ruminate and worry about what the person might be thinking.

Less obvious forms of fusion may also occur. For example, the practitioner becomes fixed on certain ideas about the direction the therapy 'should' be going at the expense of being responsive and alert to the material the person brings in the moment.

Hexaflex to Hexaflex

It can be helpful to imagine an ACT Hexaflex above the person's head, and another above our own. Each of us will have different parts of the Hexaflex dynamically positively or negatively impacting upon psychological flexibility. Hopefully, this will change for the person in a positive direction over the course of the intervention. Of course, Hexaflexes (if that is the appropriate plural!) will interact and influence *each other* as we work together with the person (or people) during each session.

Reflective practice can be helpful in considering whose Hexaflex domains are more or less enhanced or activated at any one time. For example, you may notice that you are in a session but not feeling present, and that the same is true for the other person. Once this is named, the session may be adapted to incorporate more present-moment awareness exercises, before moving on to other aspects. Equally, you may be aware that the staff team you are working with are fused on a negative attribution of the person and that you also become fused to an unhelpful thought (e.g. 'they are being obstructive'), and you may need to switch to Defusion work. Dr Russ Harris calls this 'dancing around' the Hexaflex. In reflective practice, we are considering the dance we are doing together with our person, supervisee or supporter.

Awareness of one's own limitations

There may be times where we realize that we cannot be sufficiently present for the person or their support system. While we have a job to do, we must also be realistic. We can acknowledge that the personal cannot be fully separated from the professional.

A practitioner experiencing significant personal issues, or striving to continue in work when unwell, may realize through reflection that they do not have the capacity to manage the emotional demands of a session. Rearranging the session may represent a 'towards move' on behalf of the practitioner and therefore be a better option for the person receiving therapy. Understanding one's own formulation can be helpful in such times. For example, you may be aware in a general sense that you are someone who tends to strive and struggles with self-care.

Similarly, a conscious awareness of factors that may be particularly difficult for the practitioner at certain points in life is important: for example, a referral request to support a person through grief when the practitioner has recently experienced personal bereavement. On such an occasion, perhaps alternative arrangements could be made for another clinician to pick up the case.

It is an act of compassion to self and others for practitioners to recognize when limits may be reached and to shift the focus towards reflection and self-care. It can be useful to reflect upon the motives that impact decision-making in these practical matters. The practitioner can consider their awareness of their own values and the type of practitioner they wish to be. For example, what is the driving force behind the wish to continue a session, despite awareness of poor wellbeing? Is it driven by the fear of 'letting down' the person, without due regard to the likely quality of the session? Is it a perfectionist or self-critical attitude of the practitioner? Alternatively, is the practitioner quick to cancel sessions, due to avoidance linked to anxiety about their competence? Space to reflect on one's own drivers and personal limits is important.

Acceptance

It will be important to notice when we ourselves need to 'drop the struggle'. For example, perhaps we shy away from certain topics of conversation or aspects of the ACT model, or from introducing certain exercises about which we feel less sure.

When first trained in the ACT model, one of the authors noticed their own reluctance to ask people to engage in some experiential exercises. They reflected upon why this was the case. This revealed fears about the activity not working out as planned, as well as discomfort at the idea of making the other person feel uncomfortable. Reflection upon and a willingness to move towards acceptance of the discomfort, alongside defusion from the fears, were both important to free up the practitioner to engage in the exercises that were a necessary part of the process.

Of note, some of the fears were realized! Not all of the exercises did go as planned. There was indeed nervousness on the part of the person in engaging in some of the exercises. However, we simply moved on from the exercise that did not go to plan, having normalized the experience. Other exercises went well, demonstrating and modelling to the other person that sometimes going outside of one's comfort zone pays dividends.

Values

It is important to consider one's own values as practitioners. We cannot expect people to meaningfully work on identification of their personal values if we have not done the same. Identifying our own values and therefore having a compass in our work will enhance our abilities. We recommend the completion of values exercises before delivering ACT. Use these exercises to reflect upon the type of practitioner you wish to be. This will help shape you as a practitioner, as well as giving you experience of completing the specific exercises we ask people to do.

It can also be helpful to use the Choice Point tool. Reflective space could involve reviewing the Choice Point and considering which 'towards' or 'away moves' were engaged in during sessions. It can sometimes be helpful to share our values with the people we are working with. This helps to model values work and build rapport. Establishing our own values helps to ensure we do not confuse other people's values with those of our own – a core challenge as this happens so easily with people with intellectual disabilities. We have found ongoing reflection to be important to ensure we do not steer off course and lose focus on the person's own values.

What drives our behaviour?

We should also reflect on and consider what is driving our own behaviours as practitioners. For example, are we trying to fix something unrealistically? Are we trying to be the person's rescuer? Are we trying to present ourselves as experts? Unless we make space to reflect on these issues, we could inadvertently add to the person's struggles. A benefit of using ACT is that it is so focused on person values that it can ameliorate this problem to some degree. However, an awareness of our own drivers, which may vary over time, is important in being person-centred.

> ### CASE STUDY: Regaining focus
>
> One of the authors describes an experience of working with a person who lived with her maternal uncle after her parents passed away:
>
> 'I felt a strong bond had been formed with the person, and I strived to help her to feel less lost and to have hope. However, what I was in fact doing was becoming over-involved and not being fully aware of the impact of my behaviour. Engaging in self-reflection helped me to realize that I was being driven by a desire to rescue the person. That drive was so strong that I was failing to put the person's values at the centre of the situation.
>
> 'The person themselves wanted to feel accepted by society but harboured a deep-seated fear that in fact she was not valued and even that society wished she were not alive.
>
> 'She had fears about being abandoned once her uncle was no longer alive, suggesting a value of supportiveness. This elicited strong feelings within me of a wish to rescue (which came from a value of care). This had the potential to result in my dismissing the uncle's efforts and making suggestions about activities that were not in line with the person's interests. Through reflective space I was able to recognize my lack of focus on the person's values and what was driving it. I was able to become more aligned and focused again.'

Structured reflective practice

Reflective practice is a valuable tool for enabling deeper insights and considering actions, yet as practitioners we do not always create space for it, and supporters often have even less opportunity to engage in reflective ways. It is difficult to find any existing literature on using ACT in reflective practice. However, we have engaged in the use of ACT-informed reflective space when working with supporters in some very challenging situations, to good effect. Although we do not offer a specific ACT-based reflective model or framework, we propose that it is possible (having had experience) to use the most well-established model, Gibbs' reflective framework (Gibbs,

1988), whilst exploring and integrating the following ACT elements (see also Figure 9.1):

- identification and exploration of values
- consideration of how values are and are not currently being translated to Committed Action and where the barriers may lie
- consideration of where supporters' rigidity in thinking may be impacting (e.g. 'I must always do a good job')
- analysis of how current practice can be shaped to engage in more values-based Committed Action consistent with person needs
- use of the Choice Point
- application of mindfulness approaches and exploring willingness to experience negative feelings that may arise (e.g. shame)
- introduction and application of Defusion techniques (e.g. regarding attributions and self-criticism)
- consideration of Self-as-Context issues in relation to role (e.g. exceptions to the rule 'When are you a good supporter?', what other roles you occupy, and how these link with each other).

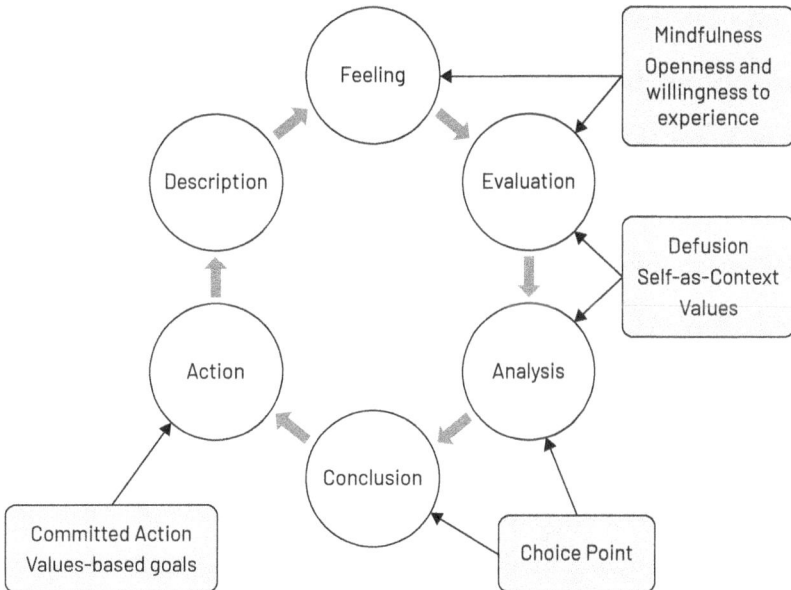

Figure 9.1 The integration of ACT principles into reflective practice, which displays the relevance of Hexaflex domains to different stages of the cycle. For example, the mindfulness domain links and may be utilized for the feelings stage of reflection, and the choice point could be an important facilitatory tool in analyzing and concluding.

SUMMARY

+ Reflective practice is an essential part of being an effective ACT practitioner.

+ Reflective practice can take place in several ways, structured and unstructured. Engaging in some form of reflective practice helps the practitioner to remain ACT consistent.

+ ACT domains can be applied to existing reflective practice models such as Gibbs' reflective cycle.

Chapter 10

USING ACT WITH THE SUPPORT SYSTEM

In this chapter, we discuss the rationale for working with the wider system. We consider where it may be appropriate, and the key principles and modes of ACT-informed systemic support. This includes consideration of the interface with indirect psychological approaches that aim to optimize the support a person receives. We describe the barriers and challenges encountered when working with systems, showing the ways in which we believe ACT can be utilized to address these challenges.

People with intellectual disabilities often rely on support from others on a daily basis. Whilst the frequency and intensity of this support will vary from person to person, it is crucial that practitioners work not only with the person, but also in a meaningful way with their support system (and sometimes solely the latter, depending on the person's level of intellectual disability and the presenting need). Every effort should be made to ensure that the individual remains at the heart of any intervention, with the utmost effort to use creative ways to empower the person to engage in a meaningful way. This includes development of communication aids if required, or collaboration with a qualified speech and language therapist where access is possible. When done well, delivering a collaborative intervention alongside supporting staff teams and/or families can help to develop a shared understanding of the person's life story and the ways in which this has shaped their current presentation. In turn, this influences the nature and quality of the support that people receive.

The context

As mentioned in Chapter 1, in the UK in the last 20 or so years there have been several horrific scandals centred around the care of people with intellectual disabilities in long-stay hospitals. One example is Winterbourne View, where significant emotional, physical and institutional abuse from support staff was uncovered. This was the catalyst for the NHS and social care 'Transforming Care Agenda' of increased scrutiny of care and hospital settings. The aim was to ensure that hospital admissions under the Mental Health Act are an absolute last resort and for as minimal a time as possible. It was at last recognized that people with intellectual disabilities were being hospitalized too often and for too long, often far away from their homes and families, and not necessarily receiving the appropriate care and treatment.

Sadly, it is both widely recognized and extremely disappointing that there is still a long way to go before the aims of the Transforming Care Agenda are achieved (Taylor, 2019). Concern around the quality of care offered to people with intellectual disabilities continues. However, the Transforming Care Agenda has led to a much greater scrutiny on the support that people with intellectual disabilities receive, which was much needed and welcomed. No one should be admitted to hospital because of a failure in the quality of support provided to them in the community.

It is well recognized that training, recruitment and having correct support packages are very important in effectively supporting someone with an intellectual disability. What often gets overlooked is the wellbeing of supporters. Their wellbeing is extremely important if people are to have good-quality/continuity of care. However, there is considerable research to evidence the high levels of stress experienced in the care sector, which has been much exacerbated by the Covid-19 pandemic (Nyashanu, Pfende & Ekpenyong, 2020). Provider services can often have a high turnover of staff. This can be devastating for the people being supported, some of whom have attachment difficulties, and all of whom rely upon a good knowledge of their needs. Some people will have had multiple placement moves, and achieving consistency and creating roots is crucial to psychological wellbeing.

Unfortunately, this does not always happen, and problems do occur, especially if a person exhibits behaviours that challenge. At its worst, a person's support can completely break down. This happened most typically due to stress and a gradual attrition of willingness on the part of those supporting the person. Sickness rates may increase where staff feel ill-equipped in their role, especially if people are displaying behavioural difficulties. Organizations may eventually serve notice on the person needing support or state that they can no longer support them. People who need support can reach a point of being admitted under the Mental Health Act due to the lack of appropriate services or emergency respite care.

There are some excellent paid supporters who intuitively know how to work well with people and who genuinely care. However, the lack of value placed on the supporting role, evidenced by the lack of requirement for qualifications and a proper career structure, means that some supporters are ill-equipped or ill-suited to the role. Furthermore, paid supporters will have some training for their roles, but it does not always focus upon the psychological needs of the people they support.

We have found that ACT can help supporters to become more in tune with their values and to work according to them. They can become more emotionally aware (and therefore less reactive) and more attuned to people's needs. A happier, more satisfied and less stressed workforce will lead to better quality of support and greater consistency, and will minimize risk of breakdown of placements.

When to consider systems work

There are many situations where we would consider the use of ACT with the wider system, for example, in cases where:

- The person relies on support from a consistent network of individuals, perhaps multidisciplinary practitioners, as well as family or paid supporters.

- The difficulties lie within the quality of the support a person receives. For example, the support system is:
    - struggling to understand the person's needs
    - not supporting the person in the most helpful or consistent way
    - having a negative, rejecting, critical or unempathic view of the person.

  This can particularly occur in more complex cases where there can be strong emotions (in turn influencing attributions) and subsequent high levels of stress and burnout.

- The person's difficulties are due to unmet social needs (e.g. insufficient number of hours of support or a lack of social opportunities). In a climate of increased cuts to public services (something we currently encounter more and more frequently in our clinical practice in the UK), some people are encouraged to use technology aids rather than paid support. These may be insufficient and can ignore the importance and need for human contact. Difficulties may then arise due to isolation and loneliness. It is established that people with intellectual disabilities tend to have far fewer friendships than people without (Taheri, Perry & Minnes, 2016), and people who experience family bereavements may find themselves increasingly lonely as they age. Far fewer people with intellectual disabilities marry or have long-term partners (McCarthy et al., 2022), and some people lose contact with their families or origin. It is not unusual for people to find that their only support network is their paid support. The use of ACT can be helpful in identifying a person's unmet needs and aiding people and their systems to think about values-based steps towards these needs being met.

- The person's difficulties are due to a lack of purpose. For example, they lack meaningful employment or valued activity. Only a small percentage of people with intellectual disabilities are thought to have paid employment. Such a scenario is not going to be addressed through individual therapy, but again, using ACT alongside the support system, and prioritizing a meaningful focus on a person's core values, can help in identifying a person's needs in this area.

- The person is being supported inappropriately (e.g. by a service provider that lacks the appropriate training and expertise).

- The degree of a person's intellectual disability means that they do not have the verbal or cognitive abilities to engage therapeutically. Therefore, a systemic approach is required.

- There is evidence that there are difficulties with the wellbeing of the support system, lack of satisfaction in their roles, and a need for opportunities for reflective space.

However, if assessment indicated that the person's difficulties were due to abuse or entirely due to a lack of sufficient support package, this may necessitate referrals elsewhere, as opposed to any kind of ACT intervention. Any social needs have to benefit from ACT principles for us to become involved.

Common challenges around support networks (and the goals)

Negative attributions (move towards positive attributions)

There is no doubt that some very good, caring and understanding supporters exist. However, when a person with intellectual disabilities presents with issues that are more complex and perhaps displaying behavioural or other difficulties, supporters will sometimes make negative attributions that can be infantilizing and dehumanizing (e.g. 'manipulating, attention-seeking, controlling'). This may be at odds with the perspective of practitioners who may know the person's history and may have developed a formulation that explains the person's behaviour from a person-centred viewpoint. For example, the formulation may indicate that the person's behaviour is a trauma response or a survival strategy that was once adaptive and necessary but no longer serves its purpose.

It can be tempting for practitioners to be critical of the lack of understanding or empathy some supporters appear to have. Instead, it is important to explore and understand why sometimes different perspectives and negative attributions exist between supporters. Failing to do so creates a battle between you as a practitioner and the relevant members of the system. This does not serve the person well and may become a perpetuating, rather than a protective, factor.

Stress (move towards healthy emotional wellbeing)

Research suggests that high stress is associated with both a lack of control in the workplace and a lack of job satisfaction (Hoboubi et al., 2017; Padmanabhan, 2021). It also shows that having the appropriate support can ameliorate stress and increase job satisfaction (Viswesvaran, Sanchez & Fisher, 1999). Supporters are often low paid and have little control over their role. Combined with the immense responsibility of supporting vulnerable people who may exhibit a range of difficulties, supporters may become more prone to reacting emotionally and unhelpfully. It is established that emotions influence attributions (and vice versa) (Zijlmans et al., 2012). ACT interventions focused on stress management can be very helpful. Remember that supporters work for long periods with people whose distress may lead to some behaviours that are highly challenging, whereas we may not. We do not know what the supporters may be having to manage, nor do we truly share that individual's lived experience. Through ACT interventions we should be seeking to find out.

CASE STUDY: Fran

Fran was a 20-year-old woman with mild intellectual disabilities and ADHD who lived with her parents. She was referred to a psychologist due to 'behaviours that challenge', but during initial assessment it was clear that there were significant difficulties in the relationship between Fran and her parents. The tension in the room was palpable. Both parents expressed frustration and desperation at Fran's behaviours (shouting, extreme anxiety about routine, separation anxiety towards Mum). Neither parent could understand why Fran was triggered by seemingly trivial things, not understanding how Fran's ADHD and learning disabilities were impacting her. Fran's dad in particular could be critical and impatient with Fran.

It was crucial to understand everyone's perspectives in this situation, making time to listen to everyone and using ACT as a practitioner to enable sitting with difficult feelings. Without doing so, it would have been likely that the psychologist would have taken a critical stance towards Fran's parents, likely resulting in disengagement. Fran described how confused she felt, how bad she felt about herself. Her mum described how little time she had for herself and how stressed she was. It was important to hold all perspectives in mind as each person's reality. While a key part of the intervention involved formulation and psychoeducation around ADHD, ACT was employed through considering Fran's values. These were kept central, even when they differed from her parents. It also included considering the origin of everyone's values (upbringing and/or the impact of neurodivergence) and encouraging the use of mindfulness when experiencing difficult emotions. It was helpful to use acceptance approaches where parents were entering into a struggle to change aspects of Fran that were unchangeable (e.g. her neurodiversity).

Othering (move towards inclusion)

The 'othering' of people with intellectual disabilities continues to occur. This may explain why what is sometimes attributed to a person with an intellectual disability would not be attributed in the same way to someone without. A lack of understanding, psychological distancing from the person, and a person's intellectual disability overshadowing other aspects of the person will lead to adopting a different, reductionist, set of rules. For example, a person self-harms in response to stressful events but does not show obvious embarrassment or shame about it. For a person with an intellectual disability, this may be seen as 'attention-seeking' rather than disinhibited, struggling to cope, or lacking the ability to consider how others may perceive their difficulties. Similarly, the person who makes false allegations (to get staff they feel unsafe with removed) becomes viewed as 'manipulative' as opposed to lacking power and control in their lives. A person who is sexually disinhibited and flirtatious may be seen as promiscuous or callous. This judgement fails to acknowledge the impact of previous sexual assaults on their behaviour or to consider how less-developed social and emotional skills affect the presentation of sexuality. At its more extreme, we have experienced supporters of people who have both significant intellectual disabilities and a history of trauma questioning why the person is struggling. They suggest that the person is being ungrateful, 'attention-seeking' or even 'spoilt'. There can be a failure to appreciate what it might be like to have an intellectual disability and all the standard experiences that can go with this, never mind the unique life experiences the person may have had. Perhaps some supporters cannot acknowledge the painful lives of the people and find ways to defend against it (an example of experiential avoidance from an ACT perspective). Others may not know what a person has experienced.

Some people have experienced multiple moves, and some have little family contact. Paid supporters may have little information about the person's history. This is an obstacle in understanding the person's life experiences and subsequent behaviours and needs. In such cases, we offer an opportunity as practitioners to collaboratively develop the narrative of a person's life. We support people to share this with relevant individuals, teams or agencies in a way that they wish.

Protecting (move towards individual empowerment)

Family members may continue to feel unresolved grief and loss about the person having an intellectual disability – the loss of the child they expected or imagined (Goldberg et al., 1995). They may feel a strong sense of protectiveness towards the person because of their disability and try to prevent the person experiencing any further distress. Understandable concern about risk may lead to over-protectiveness. For example, some people with intellectual disabilities can be overly trusting. They can be vulnerable to abuse and exploitation, and supporters can feel a strong sense of responsibility for preventing harm. While in some cases this may be completely appropriate, it can result in being risk-averse. This can lead to the person with intellectual disabilities feeling unable to engage in positive risk-taking, make their own choices or live a meaningful life.

Someone with intellectual disabilities has the right to, and indeed needs to, experience the full range of emotions and take some considered risks in the way that other people do. This may require supporters to work towards a position of acceptance around their own discomfort regarding the person with intellectual disability experiencing distress.

Limited training (move towards thorough and meaningful training)

Considering the responsibility and influence a supporter holds, it is concerning that training programmes are not more focused on addressing the psychological needs of people with intellectual disabilities. Despite the higher prevalence of mental health difficulties, mandatory training most likely will not incorporate how to help people on an emotional level. Therefore, supporters sometimes rely on their own understanding or intuition.

For some, the only experience they have had in caring might be their own children. Their intuitive response might mirror how they have responded in those situations. Many of these factors are out of our immediate control as practitioners, but we can advocate to key decision-makers for the kind of support that the person needs. We can also advocate for training and support that may help the person and their supporters. There is also the opportunity to work with supporters to enable a better understanding and to use ACT when delivering support.

Difficulties with generalizing (move towards collaborative learning of ACT skills)

A difficulty in generalizing learning has been established as a challenge for people with intellectual disabilities (Willner & Tomlinson, 2007). This may be due to cognitive challenges such as memory but may also relate to power. Some people do not have the confidence, or sense of self-efficacy, to make changes outside of the therapy setting without support. Some people show high levels of impulsivity. They will therefore find it very difficult to deploy ACT skills in relevant situations. The input of supporters is often necessary to enable generalizing and to avoid solely engaging in direct therapy that sets the person up to fail. For example, a person may learn a variety of Defusion skills in therapy and identify situations in which they wish to use them, but in the moment may forget how.

Loss of the person's voice (move towards self-advocacy and empowerment)

The vast number of people involved in the lives of a person with intellectual disabilities means that it is all too easy for the person's voice to be lost. For example, supporters may conclude that the person needs to socialize more as they have become isolated and may develop a range of activities for them to try. Has anyone asked the person if this is important to them at that moment? Do supporters know what would constitute optimal socialization for the person? An autistic person may (or may not) wish to limit their social engagement and avoid certain scenarios altogether. Does the system know what is truly important to that individual?

As we have already mentioned, supporters may not know the person's history. Time should be taken to understand what matters to them. Values-based goals should always be set alongside the person.

Person-centred plans were once popular in intellectual disability services but now seem less common. The existence of self-advocacy services can depend on the local area. There is, therefore, a need for further work in how to aid the system to maintain focus on the person in a meaningful way. Systemic formulation tools such as the CCaRM can be valuable in supporting this venture (see Chapter 2).

Job dissatisfaction (move towards pride in work and job satisfaction)

A supporter who is not working in accordance with their values is less likely to experience a sense of purpose in their work. They will feel less satisfied and more stressed. A values-based approach to a person's role can be an effective way to enhance job satisfaction. While paid supporters have job descriptions and will understand the need to ensure consistency in approaches, they will invariably have differing values in relation to their work. Is it not sensible to honour and help supporters to actualize this in their supporting role to enable better outcomes for people?

Values-matching is important. The supporters' values must not overshadow that of the individuals they support. One supporter may gain a deep sense of reward and purpose from enabling people to go outdoors and experience nature. Another will gain the most satisfaction from assisting people to become more independent and learn valuable skills.

However, this is not always adequately considered, especially in services that are struggling with staffing issues. This is a circular problem: turnover will be higher when people are not getting a sense of satisfaction from their jobs. We do not advocate that supporters develop and work towards values-based goals that are different to those of the people they are supporting, rather that organizations think more creatively about where and with whom supporters are employed to work. Matching values and interests wherever possible will lead to better outcomes.

CASE STUDY: Mismatched values

Many years ago, one of us was a volunteer in a residential home for people with intellectual disabilities:

'The mismatch between the home and me was notable: the staffing ratio was inadequate and the people residing within the home were unable to meaningfully engage in many activities. I felt little sense of value and a lack of stimulation in my role. I was motivated by being part of achieving meaningful change and improving quality of life, which was not harnessed by the organization and was stifled in the specific situation in which I worked. While a supporter has the responsibility to meet all of a person's needs, supporters need the space to express and identify these challenges within ACT-informed supervision. Once these feelings had been expressed, considering a different person/supporter arrangement would have been beneficial for me and, much more importantly, the person being supported.'

Inadequate supervision (ensure regular effective supervision)

Some paid supporters are offered inadequate opportunities for good-quality clinical and managerial supervision, if it occurs at all. In the previous case example, supervision was almost non-existent. When it occurred, it was not focused on job satisfaction or emotional content. This leaves limited opportunity to consider values in relation to the supporter role. Supervision should also create a safe space where emotions can be recognized, acknowledged and fully experienced. This includes the emotional pain that may arise when reflecting on the life history or experiences of individuals with intellectual disabilities. Additionally, supervision should allow for the expression of feelings that may emerge from the emotional demands of supporting individuals, especially when the challenges have a significant impact on the supporter's emotional and mental resources. If supporters have no space to feel and express emotions such as anger, frustration or sadness, then it will come out in some other way or at some other time.

Even when regular supervision is in place, it is often provided in a way that does not truly address the emotional impact of the complexities of the work. Often it may not include a reflective component at all. It more typically involves line-management issues or discussion on performance and can often feel like a 'tick box' exercise. Frequently, supervision does not routinely consider what truly matters to that supporter, or how their personal job satisfaction can be maximized. The ACT model can offer an opportunity for this to change.

Although family supporters may not always access the level of formal supervision that paid supporters are afforded, the principles of having a space and opportunity to share difficult feelings and reflect on the emotional impact of the caring role is really important.

Applying ACT principles to help with support systems

When working with supporters, the practitioner should gather information on the person's history to help the wider system to formulate and understand the person's perspective. Inclusion of the person should be considered at all times, in any way possible. Where this is not possible (e.g. due to the person's level of intellectual disability), alertness to values should be ensured in ways outlined in Chapter 5. This helps hold the person in mind and keeps them central to conversations.

Consent to indirect work should be sought wherever possible. Sometimes, the work will involve both indirect and direct work in tandem with, and complementing, each other. You will need to carefully consider who is involved and how: Are supporters involved in individual sessions? If so, how much? Is the person involved in supporter sessions, and again, if so, how much? What proportion of your work is with the system as opposed to with the individual? In which order will you do your interventions? All these decisions should be guided by a thorough assessment and a good formulation, and person preference where possible.

ACT-based training

Training supporters in the use of ACT approaches can make a positive difference to wellbeing and subsequent quality of support. There has been some emerging research, albeit limited, on how to utilize third-wave therapies when working with the wider system in the field of intellectual disabilities. Mindfulness-based (e.g. Singh et al., 2006) and acceptance-based interventions (Noone et al., 2006; Noone & Hastings, 2009) have had beneficial outcomes for individuals with behavioural challenges and the wellbeing of support staff.

Acceptance-based approaches have also been found to be useful in training supporters. Noone and Hastings (2009) adapted Bond and Bunce's (2000) stress workshop based on the principles of ACT and delivered this to 14 support staff at one-day workshop followed by a half-day booster session. This intervention focused both on helping staff to accept their emotions in the moment rather than trying to deny or avoid them (with the aim of helping them to be more present) and on helping staff to clarify their values and make commitments to actions more consistent with those values. Staff reported statistically significant reductions in psychological distress. We view this to be an excellent model that addresses some of the core issues we come across when working alongside supporters.

Flaxman and McIntosh (2017) have developed a four-session training model using a 'three columns' framework based on the work of Flaxman, Bond and Livheim (2013) in this area (similar to Hayes's tripartite model of 'be present, open up, do what matters'). This framework involves being: aware and active, and moving towards psychological wellbeing and life vitality. The training incorporates mindfulness exercises and psychoeducation, identification of values and action planning (and consideration of barriers), Defusion, and utilization of 'passengers on the bus', and has evidence to support its effectiveness (Towey-Swift, Lauvrud & Whittington, 2022).

Singh et al. (2006) describe a training intervention which incorporated behaviour management and a mindfulness intervention, and found that service-user aggressive behaviour reduced more dramatically, and learning was enhanced, by adding mindfulness to the behaviour training delivered to staff. Mindfulness in combination with other interventions has also been shown to help staff in combining behavioural and psychopharmacological treatment approaches for people with intellectual disabilities (Singh et al., 2003) and to improve the family-friendliness of admission teams (Singh et al., 2002). Directly training support staff in mindfulness has additionally been shown to reduce the use of physical restraints in intellectual disability-services settings (Singh et al., 2009) and to increase happiness in individuals with profound disabilities (Singh et al., 2004).

In our view, mindfulness approaches must be used judiciously since how and when they are delivered can be crucial if they are to be well received by supporters. For some, this will need to be practical, down-to-earth and clearly applicable. We recommend avoiding using the word 'mindfulness' with supporters as it may have negative connotations, and instead using terms such as 'increased awareness', 'self-awareness', 'stepping back' or 'noticing'.

However, practitioners may wish to design bespoke training, perhaps bespoke to the person. In some settings, including ours, we do not have a remit to provide general training for teams; rather, there has to be a clinical need identified through the person or people with intellectual disabilities at the heart of it. We propose that in any supporter training session it could be useful to:

- Have a specific focus on aiding staff to identify their values, how they are or could be displaying these in the workplace, how they could translate these into SMART goals (specific, measurable, achievable, relevant, timely), and how to overcome any barriers. We recommend that service managers are involved, since flexibility in organization protocols may be necessary.

- Provide psychoeducation on emotions and how to acknowledge and express emotions in a healthy way. It can be useful to devote time within a session to enabling staff teams to acknowledge and express their emotions, but it is likely that this will only be possible where there is a good relationship between practitioner and the team, and where a sense of safety is fostered.

- Encourage staff to consider the areas they have control over, and therefore can apply Committed Action (such as addressing issues in supervision; how many overtime shifts are picked up; how interactive and responsive they are with people) versus what they cannot control, and therefore need to consider acceptance approaches (such as the influence of family; the level of distress the person is experiencing due to outside events; a person's past trauma).

- Consider that where supporter sessions are focused on the person as opposed to staff wellbeing, the supporters' role in helping the person to live according to their values and goals is central.

- Teach supporters about noticing skills, particularly those more relevant to people with intellectual disabilities (e.g. soles-of-the-feet meditation described in Chapter 6).

ACT-informed positive behaviour support

Most UK providers now use and have training in the positive behaviour support (PBS) model. PBS can provide an excellent framework for providing positive support for people with complex needs. However, the quality of some PBS plans in practice can be variable. Sometimes, they can lack depth and may not sufficiently consider how supporters' own wellbeing, interactional style and cognitions, either individually or collectively, may be influencing the person. When engaging in behavioural work, seeking to establish triggers to people's behaviour is a fundamental early part of the functional analysis. However, sometimes, people will state that a person has exhibited a problematic behaviour for 'no reason at all', or that a behaviour has just 'come out of the blue', since there has been no obvious antecedent. This immediately should alert the practitioner to the possibility of an internal component, such as a cognition or memory, as the trigger (although supporters may also be missing subtle environmental factors as well). ACT incorporates the consideration of internal triggers into a behavioural framework; the challenge is in working with the support system to recognize that, just because something may not be observable, this does not mean that it isn't happening. The basis of ACT, functional contextualism, shifts the focus away from what is a problem for the supporters to considering what works and does not work for the person, as long as they do not pose risks to others or are illegal.

We suggest that ACT can be used when developing PBS plans to:

- incorporate values into plans
- apply a contextual approach
- explore carer attributions
- consider staff wellbeing
- incorporate the person's perspective into PBS workshops.

Incorporating values and skills teaching into plans

The incorporation of values into PBS plans will help to ensure a greater degree of person-centredness. Obviously, practitioners will need to make sure they have explored these values either with the person or via supporters, and we would suggest having a values-based goals section. Where a person cannot communicate or lacks insight into their values, they may be established through analysis of behaviours of concern (remembering the ACT principle 'where there is a pain there is a value'). In a functional assessment, one should always hold in mind the question 'How does this indicate what matters to the person?' We would also advocate adapting functional-analysis interview forms to include values-based questions.

Remembering the fundamental principle of 'functional contextualism', we should always be seeking to explore a person's behaviour from their point of view: Does it help the person to achieve what they want? Are we/the support system judging the behaviour through the lens of our own values? For example, supporters may identify a 'fixation with collecting leaflets' as an issue of concern, since the collection may become large and unmanageable. What is it that might be driving this behaviour? One may find that the person has a lack of a sense of predictability, and collections serve the function of enabling the person to feel more in control within a chaotic home setting. Viewed through this lens, the person's behaviour serves an important function and matters to them, and seeking to eliminate this behaviour without considering alternatives may be detrimental to the person's wellbeing. Supporters may need to recognize that predictability for this person is an important value, and whilst they may disagree and view it as problematic, it is not person-centred to seek to eliminate the behaviour.

In some ways, this is a standard approach within PBS, in that determining the function of the behaviour and looking for more suitable alternatives always occur; the difference is that when considering through an ACT lens you are looking not only at the activity but also at the value that underpins it, which then opens up more options. For example, leaflets may play a less important role for the person and therefore be more manageable if there is an increase in other routines in their life.

Where appropriate, include explicit elements in relation to ACT-related skills that the person can be offered the opportunity to learn. These should be relevant to the things that the person may be struggling with: for example, dropping-anchor skills for people struggling with anger and anxiety coping skills, or Defusion skills for someone who is becoming frustrated due to dwelling on particular thoughts or memories. It is helpful to be explicit about the skills the person will be offered the opportunity to develop, and how the person can be supported to practise and use the skills. In addition to specific skills, exercises like the lifeline task can be used to work with the person about what information about them they would like to have in their PBS plans, and to help develop a coherent sense of self. An example of an ACT-informed PBS plan:

Name:
Date of birth:
Address:

What is important to Adam and why? (*'The things that are important to me, because...'*)
'My family, going to the gym, my pet lizard, having a takeaway every weekend; wearing designer clothes.'

What values are important to the service, and to you as a staff team when working with Adam? (*'The things that are important to my team when they support me'*)
Having the resources to help Adam to do the things that are important to him: e.g. enough staff on shift so that we can support trips to the gym, and visits to family; and having money accessible and arranged in advance to pay for activities, such as the bus fare to the gym and take-aways at the weekend. Also having regular breaks.

What are Adam's strengths? (*'My strengths, positive things about me, things that I am really good at'*)
Adam is a very kind person. Adam is great at playing pool. Adam is very caring, especially towards his family and pet lizard. Adam has great jokes and makes people laugh often.

What behaviours does Adam display, and what does he want to achieve through them? (*'When I am distressed, sometimes I may... Often this is because I hope to.../I was feeling...'*)
Adam sometimes runs away from staff. Adam sometimes becomes angry and breaks items of property around the house such as mugs or tele-visions. When this happens, Adam has often been feeling lonely and isolated; Adam may have felt that he had been ignored and runs away in order to guarantee one-to-one time with staff. In the past, when Adam has thrown items in the home such as mugs, staff have heard the mug smash and run to his flat to check everything was okay.

Early signs of distress ('*The things that people may notice me doing when I am starting to feel distressed*')
Adam repeatedly opening and closing the cupboard doors in his flat, and pacing around his flat (staff may hear his footsteps walking back and forth in his flat above the office). Adam talking out loud to himself. Adam starting to walk faster when out and about with staff, gradually getting ahead of supporters and peers.

What makes Adam distressed? ('*The things that make me feel distressed/angry/"wound up"*') [*Use individual's preferred terminology*]
'Feeling left out. People ignoring me. Staff being on their phones – they're meant to be looking after me. Other people talking to my staff and taking them away from me when I want to talk to them.'

Proactive strategies (to use at baseline) ('*Ways that people can help me before I get worked up*')
'At the start of the week, let me know who is on shift each day (this can be in the form of a notice board outside the staff office); if anyone calls in sick or won't be in work, update the board so that I know who will be coming to support me.

'Every morning after breakfast, come and chat to me about plans for the day. Talk through the things we will be doing and be clear about when I will have some uninterrupted one-to-one time with staff, just to talk about the things on my mind. Sometimes, I may not have anything to talk about, but please still come and see me so we can spend some time together. This helps me feel as though I am important and valued and that somebody cares.'

Strategies to use when Adam is becoming distressed ('*Things people can do to support me when I am becoming wound up – It can also be helpful here to see the difference between 'the things I can do to help myself' and 'the things other people can do to help me' when I am becoming distressed*')

'If I notice I am becoming worked up, I can:

- drop anchor, check in with myself and notice five things I can see, hear, smell, taste and feel
- take some deep breaths
- put my favourite music on

- look at photos of my family.'

'When I am becoming worked up, other people can help me by:

- knocking on my door and asking me if I would like to talk (ideally, this would have happened before I reached the point of distress)
- directing me to my sensory box, which includes different soothing activities I can do when I feel worked up
- sitting down with me and doing some noticing exercises, checking-in together, and working out a plan for "now and next"
- reminding me of how far I have come.'

Reactive strategies ('The things people can do to help me if I have become distressed')

- Make sure that the area is safe and remove items that I may hurt myself on.
- Allow me time to 'calm down' (I'm happy for my staff to use this phrase for me as it helps me, but I know that this phrase may wind other people up).
- Let me know that you are here to help me and can chat to me when I feel ready.
- Avoid getting into an argument/confrontation whilst I am feeling angry; this is not helpful and just winds me up even more.

Supporter wellbeing strategies ('Ways that the people who support me can look after themselves too') [Include staff use of values-based supervision, debriefing, staff coping strategies]

- Regular supervision with a qualified professional and opportunities to talk about the emotional impact of some of the feelings conjured up through work with Adam.
- Ensuring regular breaks during shifts; remaining mindful of number of hours worked, even if the team are short staffed, knowing it is okay to have time off and work towards a healthy work/life balance.
- Trying hard to attend the regular mindfulness sessions offered within the team.

Applying a contextual approach

A cornerstone of the ACT model is the universality of human suffering and the contextual approach. Good-quality PBS plans should not locate 'problems' within the person. Using the principles of ACT, it can be helpful to include phrases such as 'like many people: for example, 'Like many people, David can feel frustrated at times, and he shows this by...'.

PBS can reduce blame by being contextual. Whenever a difficulty is discussed, try to note in what circumstances these difficulties occur: for example, 'Xang can struggle with feeling anxious in busy places when he is with unfamiliar staff members'. This is certainly not a principle that is unique to ACT-informed PBS but having an ACT mindset when completing plans can help ensure adherence to these principles.

Exploring carer attributions

Are there aspects of language and relational framing that need to be worked on? For example, has the supporter formed a view that the person with intellectual disabilities is 'manipulative'? Or is the carer holding a rigid view of themselves in their workplace, for example:

- 'I must never have an incident with any of the people I support.'
- 'I am not here to get hit.' (This understandable view does get expressed by some supporters who have recently experienced behaviours that challenge for the first time.)

Again, the consideration of attributions of supporters is not new. In ACT work it is considered in terms of relational frames and ways in which to reduce psychological inflexibility, in this case, via Defusion. It can sometimes be difficult to alter supporter attributions, but what can be worked on is encouraging supporters to notice and defuse from them.

Considering staff wellbeing

Many PBS practitioners will (and should) already consider supporter stress and wellbeing as part of their assessment. However, the ACT model offers a different way of doing so. Hexaflex skills can be developed through forums that bring together the wider system in order to consider behaviours of concern by devoting a part of the session to considering staff needs. We would suggest referring to the subsection dealing with stress earlier in this chapter, to explore this in more depth.

Incorporating the person's perspective into PBS workshops

PBS plans should never be developed in a 'done to' way – that is, the practitioner completing an assessment, writing a plan and giving this to those involved, with an expectation that it will be followed. We know this does not work. Plans must be developed collaboratively with everyone involved, and we would recommend holding 'PBS workshops' in order to do so, especially with more complex cases. In a study of the experiences of facilitators and participants of PBS workshops for complex cases (Tomlinson, 2007), it was found that a number of factors were considered important and needed consideration when working with the system to develop PBS plans:

- having a strong relationship (akin to the therapeutic relationship) between facilitator and participants
- having an environment of safety and trust
- having a sense of collaboration.

When facilitating such workshops, we recommend incorporating ACT approaches.

The prosocial model

The prosocial model (Atkins, Wilson & Hayes, 2019)[1] offers an approach to group working that has contextual and behavioural principles underlying it, focused on enhancing group ability to 'move flexibly in valued directions despite changing contexts'. It is based on aligning individual and group interests and reinforcing co-operative behaviours. We are social beings, and, done right, there is power in groups acting as a single 'organism'.

Principles of the prosocial model are (Ostrom, 1990, cited in Atkins et al., 2019):

- shared identity and purpose
- fair distribution of contributions and benefits
- fair and inclusive decision-making
- monitoring of agreed behaviours
- graduated responding to helpful and unhelpful behaviour
- fast and fair conflict resolution
- authority to self-govern
- appropriate relations with other groups.

---

1   The prosocial model combines ACT and multi-level selection theory (Wilson & Sober, 1994) with Nobel Laureate Elinor Ostrom's core design principles for effective group-level processes (Ostrom, 2012, 2015).

The prosocial model strongly emphasizes enhancing the ability of participants to take the perspectives of others, empathize, regulate emotions and
understand goals, values and needs to achieve change. This requires an
essential phase of inner work where participants learn how to become more
psychologically flexible.

Since practitioners in learning disability services are often working with
systems, whether this is through multidisciplinary teams, supporters or others, the prosocial model can be usefully applied. For example, developing
a PBS plan is not simply a matter of establishing functions and making
recommendations; parties will have different perspectives, and there will
be different relational dynamics at play within the system, particularly in
complex cases.

- The first stage in the prosocial process is to build a context for change:
  this may be the stage where values-based goals are identified as a
  group.
- The second stage is building a sense of shared vision identity and
  purpose: this is also where shared values can be identified.
- The third stage is exploring aspects of prosocial governance: this is
  where the group explores how it can work together to be allies, and
  determines its goals, and here Ostrom's (2012, 2015) principles can
  be applied. The group uses the psychological flexibility skills built
  earlier to turn towards the question of how to achieve its vision. The
  process helps to resist rigidity and create space for new understanding
  and is a useful model to consider when engaging in the process of
  developing a PBS plan or engaging in other types of systems work.

Using the Choice Point with the wider system

The Choice Point is a useful tool to use with supporters, whether in supervision, reflective practice, training or in staff/family sessions. Supporters
should be encouraged to develop values-based goals in respect of the people they support. Whilst there is a permeable home/work boundary (and we
should explore areas where supporters' home lives may impact upon work),
the focus upon non-work-related issues should be avoided. This needs to
be a clear boundary at the outset. The supporting role must be kept central.
Similar to when using the Choice Point directly with people with intellectual
disabilities, consider the systemic factors that are facilitators or barriers to
change as well as individual factors.

Too often, organizations adopt a blame approach to staff stress without
considering the organization's role within it. For example, the emphasis can
often be more upon the individual developing coping strategies for their

stress, rather than considering how the wider system may change to support the individual.

It can also be helpful to consider how a person's Choice Point interacts with that of their supporters. Doing so may highlight differences and similarities between the person with intellectual disabilities and their supporters. This will therefore increase awareness, encouraging opportunities where values may be similar, and respect where they differ.

The Choice Point can also be used as part of reflective practice sessions. This can be done in exactly the same way as when engaging in therapy, except that here the focus is on matters relating to the people they support. First, establish the supporter's values and how these can be translated to values-based goals. Then go on to consider where the supporter may feel triggered by the person, and how the supporter may make 'towards moves' rather than 'away moves'. An example is provided in the following case study of Harry, with Figure 10.1 summarizing his Choice Point, developed through group reflective practice sessions facilitated by a psychologist.

CASE STUDY: Harry

Harry was a 50-year-old man who had worked as a paid supporter for many years. He had been feeling unmotivated and stressed due to changes in a person's presentation (increased aggression) with an unclear cause.

Through regular ACT-based reflective practice sessions, Harry was able to identify that he was having many negative thoughts towards himself ('I am terrible at my job', 'other people can cope better than me'), leading to emotion-/stress-driven attributions towards the person ('they are doing it on purpose', 'they don't like me', 'they're just doing it for attention').

Adding to this, Harry experienced guilt about his negative thoughts about the person (value: kindness or harmony) and frustrated at being unable to make a difference to the person's situation (value: contribution). His overwork due to short staffing reduced time with his family or on his hobbies, both important values. Through the reflective sessions, Harry became more aware. He began to establish goals he could set for himself, such as 'say no to extra shifts', 'take regular annual leave', 'schedule in regular time with his family', and 'arrange some photography classes'. He also learned Defusion skills, ('notice the inner critic') and acceptance ('notice the feeling and let it be there').

Harry was able to ask for increased supervision with his manager. In supervision, they identified times when Harry could work with other people to enable them to achieve their goals (value: contribution). Over time, Harry began to feel more satisfied with his job again and less stressed. He was more able to cope with the person's behaviour and be less reactive to it.

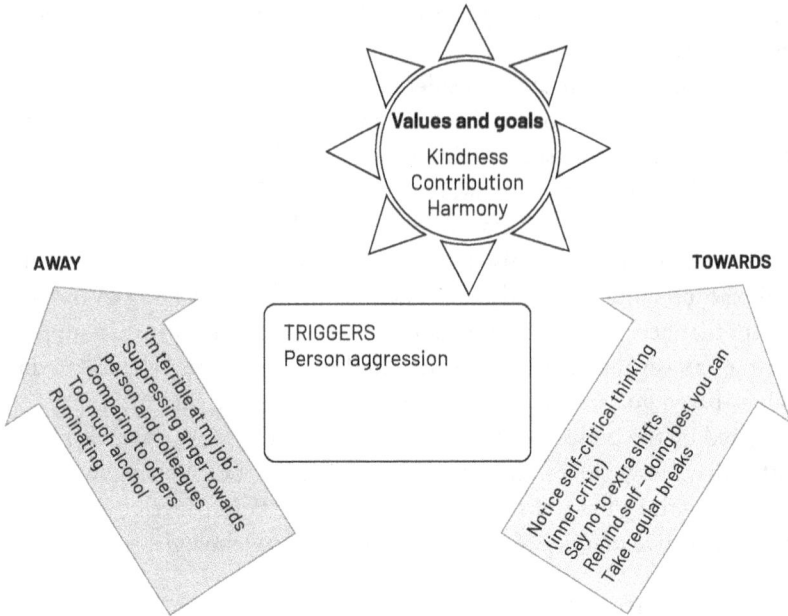

Figure 10.1 *Using the Choice Point with supporters*

Trauma-informed principles

We have already stated that the experience of trauma is far higher for someone with an intellectual disability. Therefore, as a practitioner, you *will* be working with traumatized individuals on a regular basis. You may not always be aware of it. Trauma symptoms in people with intellectual disabilities are underrecognized, and it is not always possible to know a person's full history.

This can create vicarious trauma, sometimes referred to as 'compassion fatigue' (Jimenez et al., 2021). Supporters may also have their own traumatic experiences, which can have an impact in the workplace, especially if required to simultaneously manage the trauma responses of the people they support.

The importance of trauma-informed healthcare has been increasingly recognized in recent years. Key trauma-informed principles include safety, trustworthiness, peer support, collaboration, empowerment, and cultural, historical and gender acknowledgements (Centre for Substance Abuse Treatment, 2014).

It is beyond the scope of this book to go into this in depth. We recommend as further reading the edited book *Trauma and Intellectual Disability: Acknowledgement, Identification and Intervention* (Beail, Frankish & Skelly, 2021), which deals specifically with trauma and people with intellectual disabilities.

We believe that the use of ACT with the wider support network with respect to trauma can be useful because:

- *Working with trauma is a particularly emotive area*: Whether above or below conscious awareness, there are more likely to be transference reactions and relational difficulties where someone has experienced trauma. The ability to sit with and hear the painful experiences someone has had requires willingness to experience difficult emotions, which is a central tenet of ACT. Many people with intellectual disabilities have had repeated and horrific traumatic experiences; hearing their stories or simply unconsciously feeling their pain can be very difficult.

- *Trauma may relate to attachment*: People with intellectual disabilities are more likely to have experienced disrupted attachments for a number of reasons including:
  - parental difficulties bonding with their child caused by differences in attachment care-seeking behaviours in the infant (e.g. smiling or crying less) leading to a different dynamic
  - higher prevalence of abuse and neglect
  - behavioural difficulties causing higher stress levels for parents.
  This is sometimes referred to as relational or complex trauma.

Many of the challenges to living a good life and enjoying good mental health are interpersonal in nature. For example, having a lack of a social network is a key predictor of poor mental health. Bear in mind a person's learning history in relating to other humans, not just on a cognitive level but also in learned responses and unconscious patterns of interacting. Bear in mind also how different social situations affect the person's physiological reactions because of their learning history. Attachment styles of both the person and individuals in the wider system can be overlooked yet so significant. This is especially the case where someone has experienced early childhood trauma. The system needs to understand the relational dynamics in order to consider new ways of relating.

Attachment style may be considered an example of psychological inflexibility. Perhaps at the time the attachment style of the child was adaptive but has since become maladaptive. Enhancing psychological flexibility, whether this be for the person or the wider system, will enable new relational patterns to occur that are more aligned with the person's values. New attachment styles and problem-solving abilities can thus be developed and nurtured.

Supervision and appraisals for supporters

Supervision can take many forms, ranging from didactic to reflective. Reflective supervision is much less used and yet is very important in enhancing self-awareness and reducing stress. We recommend integrating ACT principles into supporters' supervision and appraisals (this can also be used for practitioners) by having a focus on values, providing space for acknowledging feelings that arise when at work, having values-driven goals (perhaps in addition to the organization's values) and even using the Choice Point. Here is an example of an ACT-based supervision record.

Name: Jane Jones

Values-based goals: Curiosity/learning, variety/stimulation, peacefulness, team working, adventure, keeping fit, being understanding.

Stressors: High noise levels, lack of clarity, boredom, being enclosed for long periods, routine.

Service/staff agreement: Jane to be allocated to outdoor activities with people where possible; to avoid working with noisy people where feasible; to be given regular, clear feedback on performance; and to be ensured time for learning more about topics of interest (autism/trauma).

Review of week
Date of supervision: 22/03/23
Values-based achievements in past week: Took people to a variety of outdoor activities, attended training on autism, week has been varied.

Challenges: Stressful day on Tuesday due to person incident where trigger was unclear. Jane was concerned that she should have prevented it.

Emotions experienced: At the time, high anxiety as incident occurred in public. Later, guilt and frustration at not having prevented it. Anger towards colleague Fran, who was not supportive.

Review of:
Fusion/Defusion: I noticed strong thoughts at the time that Fran was lazy. Later, I had thoughts that I was unkind for thinking this about her. I was highly fused to these and this created anxiety. Whilst less present

now, I am encouraging myself to notice the thoughts when they come up and recognize they are only thoughts. Doing this is making me wonder if she may have been afraid or not confident.

Noticing: I supressed my anger towards Fran due to guilt, but it didn't go away. I am now acknowledging it.

Views of self: I noticed myself thinking I was unkind and tried hard to remember times where I have been kind.

Acceptance: I realize that a range of difficult feelings can come up in an incident. This is okay.

Values-based actions: My feelings caused me to avoid Fran for a while, which made things worse. I reflected on how my annoyance towards her was because of my wish to do the best for my person.

Learning: Acknowledge feelings when they are there, don't get into 'shoulds': It's normal to find an incident difficult and for difficult feelings to come up. Avoiding Fran will make things worse. Talk openly to her about the incident.

How others can help: Some time away from the person/Fran to debrief immediately.

Morris and Bilich-Eric (2017) have developed an ACT-informed supervision model named SHAPE: Supervision values; Hold stories lightly; Analysis of function; Perspective-taking and Experiential methods. Whilst this paper describes some extremely useful ways in which to do ACT-based supervision, we believe that having a structure such as that displayed in the ACT-informed supervision record helps the practitioner to adhere to the model, in a flexible manner of course.

Supporting direct work

As we have previously mentioned, because people with intellectual disabilities often having difficulties with generalization (Willner & Tomlinson, 2007), supporters can be crucial in assisting people to utilize what takes place in ACT-based therapy sessions. To achieve this, supporters should have sufficient knowledge of the ACT model. Practitioners must devote enough time to ensuring supporters fully understand both the model and their role in assisting people to apply ACT in their daily lives.

Do not overestimate supporters' knowledge of therapy models or principles. Ensure the basics are covered. Do not assume an understanding of the links between thoughts, feelings and behaviours. Even some words like *anxiety* may need to be defined – it is not an everyday term for some. If supporters do not fully understand the ACT model, there is a danger an inconsistent message will be given to the person they are supporting, and generalization may not occur.

The education of supporters in the ACT model can include attending training sessions, providing leaflets or recommending the supporter or organization purchases an easy-to-read book on ACT. We recommend *ACT Made Simple* (2019), *The Happiness Trap* (2007) and *The Illustrated Happiness Trap* (2014), all by Russ Harris.

Using ACT in teams

Practitioners who work within teams (e.g. in health and/or social care) can use ACT principles in team working. This could be through delivering training; integrating ACT principles into consultations, supervisions or reflective practice sessions; and shaping the team's mission statements or aims and objectives, for example by encouraging people to identify their values.

Most teams of professionals supporting people with intellectual disabilities are filled with caring, giving people. Sadly, in the UK, levels of stress and burnout in health and social care staff are high. UK health and social-care public services have seen an upsurge in referrals since the Covid-19 pandemic, without a commensurate increase in resources. In order to retain what are often excellent employees, we argue that the onus is on the employer and managers in the system to ensure staff are offered adequate support. The use of ACT-based reflection and supervision offers one way to support team members in feeling satisfied in their jobs, which will subsequently have an effect on staff retention and sickness.

SUMMARY

* There are a range of challenges faced by supporters. Given their central importance in the lives of people with intellectual disabilities it is crucial that practitioners intervene at the systemic level if indicated.

- ACT can be applied to many systemic interventions, including: the integration of ACT principles into PBS plans, training, supervision, using the Choice Point, and aiding supporters in generalization of skills. In particular, the consideration of supporters' values, and how these interact with those of the person, can be very helpful.

CONCLUSION: WHERE DO WE GO FROM HERE?

We are pleased to see a small but growing community of ACT practitioners in the UK, working with both the general population and with people with intellectual disabilities. This has not yet translated into a great deal of research among the intellectual disability practice field, but we hope that this will come in time.

We would, of course, love to see ACT being used to a greater degree in practice alongside people with intellectual disabilities and their supporters. It is wonderful that ACT is now taught on some professional courses, such as some doctoral courses in clinical psychology. There are certainly pockets of ACT-based work occurring all over UK intellectual disability services and perhaps in other countries.

High-quality research into ACT for people with intellectual disabilities is essential in order for ACT to be considered as an evidence-based treatment for people with intellectual disabilities. Despite the evidence base only now emerging, there has been significant progress over the last few decades. We hope that the ACT-ID community can continue to fly the flag for this potentially pivotal approach, working towards a focus on values at the heart of therapeutic intervention for people with intellectual disabilities.

We would love to see a greater emphasis on using ACT for people with intellectual disabilities, which can be achieved through word-of-mouth, research and local/national ACT special interest groups (please contact the authors should you be interested in joining ours!), networking, and sharing our stories of successes and challenges along the way.

We would implore you to get involved and not to be afraid to give it a go. Really immerse yourself in the model and use ACT in your everyday life – you may just be amazed at the results and subsequent shift in aspects of both your personal and professional life! If you haven't done so already, access some high-quality training. Surround yourself with other people who love ACT for people with ID (either in person, or via the wonders of the virtual world). Don't be afraid to conjure up creative research ventures and do your utmost to find a way to follow these through. Always think outside of the box, challenge those boundaries, and be brave and bold to overcome barriers. Find the spark that fuels your passion and the things that truly matter, and maintain the person at the heart of the work you do, always.

We leave you with two final quotes from Steve Hayes (2011) that should be kept in mind in all of your work:

The goal is not to fix people, but to empower them.

The process of living is like taking a very important road trip.
The destination may be important, but the journey experienced
day to day and week to week is what is invaluable.

We hope that we have helped to empower *you* through this book. We wish you the very best on your journey, and in supporting others on their own journeys.

References

Allen, D., James, W., Evans, J., Hawkins, S. & Jenkins, R. (2005). Positive behavioural support: Definition, current status and future directions. *Tizard Learning Disability Review, 10*(2), 4–11.

Allez, K., Cappleman, R., Chinn, D. & Dodd, K. (2023). *Psychologists Promoting and Supporting the Physical Health of People with Learning Disabilities: Guidance.* Leicester: British Psychological Society.

American Psychological Association (2018). Suggestibility. *APA Dictionary of Psychology.* https://dictionary.apa.org/suggestibility

Association for Contextual Behavioral Science. (n.d.). Acceptance and Commitment Therapy (ACT). https://contextualscience.org/act

Atkins, P. W., Wilson, D. S. & Hayes, S. C. (2019). *Prosocial: Using Evolutionary Science to Build Productive, Equitable, and Collaborative Groups.* New Harbinger.

Audit Commission. (1986). *Making a Reality of Community Care.* Audit Commission for Local Authorities in England and Wales. HMSO.

Baddeley, A. (1986). *Working Memory.* Clarendon Press/Oxford Press.

Banks, R. & Bush, A. (2016). *Challenging Behaviour: A Unified Approach: Update.* Clinical and service guidelines for supporting children, young people and adults with intellectual disabilities who are at risk of receiving abusive or restrictive practices. Report from the Faculties of Intellectual Disability of the Royal College of Psychiatrists and the British Psychological Society on behalf of the Learning Disabilities Professional Senate.

Barnes-Holmes, Y., Hayes, S. C., Barnes-Holmes, D. & Roche, B. (2001). Relational frame theory: A post-Skinnerian account of human language and cognition. *Advances in Child Development and Behavior, 28,* 101–138. doi:10.1016/s0065-2407(02)80063-5

Barrowcliff, A. L. & Evans, G. A. (2015). EMDR treatment for PTSD and intellectual disability: A case study. *Advances in Mental Health and Intellectual Disabilities, 9*(2), 90–98.

Beail, N., Warden, S., Morsey, K. & Newman, D. W. (2005). A naturalistic evaluation of the effectiveness of psychodynamic psychotherapy with adults with intellectual disabilities. *Journal of Applied Research in Intellectual Disabilities. 18,* 245–251.

Beail, N., Frankish, P. & Skelly, A. (2021). *Trauma and Intellectual Disability: Acknowledgement, Identification and Intervention.* Pavilion.

Beck, A. T. (1976). *Cognitive Therapy and the Emotional Disorders.* International Universities Press.

Beck, J. S. (1995). *Cognitive Therapy: Basics and Beyond.* Guilford Press.

Bender, M. (1993). The unoffered chair: The history of therapeutic disdain towards people with a learning difficulty. *Clinical Psychology Forum, 28*(54),7–12. British Psychological Society.

Biglan, A. & Hayes, S. C. (1996). Should the behavioral sciences become more pragmatic? The case for functional contextualism in research on human behavior. *Applied and Preventive Psychology, 5*(1), 47–57.

Biglan, A., Hayes, S. C. & Pistorello, J. (2008). Acceptance and commitment: Implications for prevention science. *Prevention Science, 9*, 139–152.

Boddington, E., Pethe-Kulkarni, A., O'Brien, C. & Johnson, G. (2018). The development and adaption of an acceptance and commitment based therapy group for people with learning disabilities. *Bulletin of the Faculty for People with Intellectual Disabilities, 16*(1), 19–25.

Bond, F. W. & Bunce, D. (2000). Mediators of change in emotion-focused and problem-focused worksite stress management interventions. *Journal of Occupational Health Psychology, 5*(1), 156–163.

Boulton, N. E., Williams, J. & Jones, R. S. P. (2018a). Could participant-produced photography augment therapeutic interventions for people with intellectual disabilities? A systematic review of the available evidence. *Journal of Intellectual Disabilities, 22*(1), 74–95. doi:10.1177/1744629516663027

Boulton, N. E., Williams, J. & Jones, R. S. P. (2018b). Intellectual disabilities and ACT: Feasibility of a photography-based values intervention. *Advances in Mental Health and Intellectual Disabilities, 12*(1), 11–21. doi:10.1108/AMHID-07-2017-0028

Boulton, N. E., Williams, J. & Jones, R. S. P. (2020). 'Catching what matters': A values-based ACT intervention for people with intellectual disabilities. *Bulletin of the Faculty for People with Intellectual Disabilities, 18*(2). doi:10.53841/bpsfpid.2020.18.2.20

Bozarth, J. (2007). Unconditional Positive Regard. In M. Cooper, M. O'Hara, P. F. Schmid & G. Wyatt (Eds.), *The Handbook of Person-centred Psychotherapy and Counselling* (pp.182–193). Palgrave Macmillan/Springer Nature.

British Psychological Society. (2015). *Guidance on the Assessment and Diagnosis of Intellectual Disabilities in Adulthood.* BPS.

Brown, F. J. & Hooper, S. (2009). Acceptance and commitment therapy (ACT) with a learning disabled young person experiencing anxious and obsessive thoughts. *Journal of Intellectual Disabilities, 13*(3), 195–201.

Bruce, M., Collins, S., Langdon, P., Powlitch, S. & Reynolds, S. (2010). Does training improve understanding of core concepts in cognitive behaviour therapy by people with intellectual disabilities? A randomized experiment. *British Journal of Clinical Psychology, 49*(1), 1–13.

Byrne, G. & O'Mahony, T. (2020). Acceptance and commitment therapy (ACT) for adults with intellectual disabilities and/or autism spectrum conditions (ASC): A systematic review. *Journal of Contextual Behavioral Science, 18*, 247–255.

Byrne, M., Higgins, A. & De Vries, J. (2023). Cognitive dissonance and depression: A qualitative exploration of a close relationship. *Current Research in Social Psychology, 32*, Article 1.

Campbell, D. (2013). Normative Data. In: F. R. Volkmar (Ed.) *Encyclopedia of Autism Spectrum Disorders.* Springer.

Carr, E. G., Horner, R. H., Turnbull, A. P. et al. (1999). *Positive behavioral support for people with developmental disabilities: A research synthesis.* American Association on Mental Retardation. Washington, DC.

Carr, E. G., Dunlap, G., Horner, R. H., Koegel, R. L. et al. (2002). Positive behavior support: Evolution of an applied science. *Journal of Positive Behavior Interventions, 4*(1), 4–16. doi:10.1177/109830070200400102

Center for Substance Abuse Treatment (US). (2014). Trauma-Informed Care in Behavioral Health Services. Rockville (MD): Substance Abuse and Mental Health Services Administration (US). *Treatment Improvement Protocol (TIP) Series,* 57. Available from: https://www.ncbi.nlm.nih.gov/books/NBK207201/

Chinn, D., Abraham, E., Burke, C. & Davies, J. (2014). *IAPT and Learning Disabilities.* Research Report. King's College and Foundation for People with Learning Disabilities, London.

Clapton, N. E., Williams, J. & Jones, R. S. (2018). The role of shame in the development and maintenance of psychological distress in adults with intellectual disabilities: A narrative review and synthesis. *Journal of Applied Research in Intellectual Disabilities, 31*(3), 343–359.

Clapton, N. E., Williams, J., Griffith, G. M. & Jones, R. S. (2018). 'Finding the person you really are… on the inside': Compassion focused therapy for adults with intellectual disabilities. *Journal of Intellectual Disabilities, 22*(2), 135–153.

Cooper, S.-A., Smiley, E., Morrison, J., Williamson, A. & Allan, L. (2007). Mental ill-health in adults with intellectual disabilities: Prevalence and associated factors. *British Journal of Psychiatry, 190*(1), 27–35.

Cooper, S.-A., Hughes-McCormack, L., Greenlaw, N. & McConnachie, A. (2018). Management and prevalence of long-term conditions in primary health care for adults with intellectual disabilities compared with the general population: A population-based cohort study. *Journal of Applied Research in Intellectual Disabilities, 31*, 68–81.

Dagnan, D., Chadwick, P. & Proudlove, J. (2000). Toward an assessment of suitability of people with mental retardation for cognitive therapy. *Cognitive Therapy and Research, 24*, 627–636. doi:10.1023/A:1005531226519

Dagnan, D., Taylor, L. & Burke, C. K. (2023). Adapting cognitive behaviour therapy for people with intellectual disabilities: An overview for therapist working in mainstream or specialist services. *The Cognitive Behaviour Therapist, 16*, e3. doi:10.1017/S1754470X22000587

Delap, L. (2023). Slow workers: Labelling and labouring in Britain, c.1909–1955. *Social History of Medicine, 37*(1), 160–182. doi:10.1093/shm/hkad043

Department of Health. (2012). *Transforming Care: A National Response to Winterbourne View.*

Department of Health and Social Care. (2022). *An action plan to strengthen community support for people with a learning disability and autistic people, and reduce reliance on mental health inpatient care.*

Dion, J., Paquette, G., Tremblay, K. N., Collin-Vezina, D. & Chabot, M. (2018). Child maltreatment among children with intellectual disability in the Canadian incidence study. *American Journal of Intellectual and Developmental Disabilities, 123*(2), 176–188.

Division of Clinical Psychology (2011). *Guidelines for Clinical Psychology Services.* British Psychological Society.

Dunlop, B. J. & Lea, J. (2023). 'It's not just in my head': An intersectional, social and systems-based framework in gender and sexuality diversity. *Psychology and Psychotherapy: Theory, Research and Practice, 96*(1), 1–15.

Emerson, E. & Baines, S. (2010). *The Estimated Prevalence of Autism among Adults with Learning Disabilities in England.* Improving Health and Lives: Learning Disabilities Observatory, Durham.

Felitti, V. J., Anda R. F., Nordenberg, D., Edwards, V. et al. (1998). Relationship of childhood abuse and household dysfunction to many of the leading causes of death in adults. *American Journal of Preventive Medicine, 14*(4), 245–258.

Felver, J. C., Clawson, A. J., Ash, T. L., Martens, B. K., Wang, Q. & Singh, N. N. (2022). Meta-analysis of mindfulness-based program 'Soles of the Feet' for disruptive behaviors. *Behavior Modification, 46*(6), 1488–1516.

Festinger, L. (1962). *A Theory of Cognitive Dissonance.* Stanford University Press.

Finlay, L. (2008). A dance between the reduction and reflexivity: Explicating the 'phenomenological psychological attitude'. *Journal of Phenomenological Psychology, 39*(1), 1–32.

Finlay, W. M. & Lyons, E. (2001). Methodological issues in interviewing and using self-report questionnaires with people with mental retardation. *Psychological Assessment, 13*(3), 319.

Flaxman, P. E., Bond, F. W. & Livheim, F. (2013). *The Mindful and Effective Employee: An Acceptance and Commitment Therapy Training Manual for Improving Well-Being and Performance.* New Harbinger.

Ge, B. H. & Yang, F. (2023). Transcending the self to transcend suffering. *Frontiers in Psychology, 7*(14), 1113965. doi:10.3389/fpsyg.2023.1113965

Gibbs, G. (1988). *Learning by Doing: A guide to teaching and learning methods.* Oxford: Further Education Unit, Oxford Polytechnic.

Gilbert, P. (2000). Social Mentalities: Internal 'Social' Conflicts and the Role of Inner Warmth and Compassion in Cognitive Therapy. In P. Gilbert & K. G. Bailey (Eds.), *Genes on the Couch: Explorations in Evolutionary Psychotherapy* (pp.118–150). Routledge.

Gilbert, P. & Choden (2013). *Mindful Compassion*. Hachette UK.

Goldberg, D., Magrill, L., Hale, J., Damaskinidou, K., Paul, J. & Tham, S. (1995). Protection and loss: Working with learning-disabled adults and their families. *Journal of Family Therapy, 17*(3), 263–280.

Gore, N. J. & Hastings, R. P. (2016). Mindfulness and Acceptance-based Therapies. In N. Beal (Ed.), *Psychological Therapies and People Who Have Intellectual Disabilities* (pp.11–19), British Psychological Society.

Greenhill, B. & Whitehead, R. (2010). Promoting service user inclusion in risk assessment and management: A pilot project developing a human rights-based approach. *British Journal of Learning Disabilities, 39*, 277–283.

Griffith, G. M. & Hastings, R. P. (2014). 'He's hard work, but he's worth it': The experience of caregivers of individuals with intellectual disabilities and challenging behaviour: A meta-synthesis of qualitative research. *Journal of Applied Research in Intellectual Disabilities, 27*(5), 401–419.

Gudjonsson, G. H. & Henry, L. (2003). Child and adult witnesses with intellectual disability: The importance of suggestibility. *Legal and Criminological Psychology, 8*(2), 241–252.

Hall, J. C., Jobson, L. & Langdon, P. E. (2014). Measuring symptoms of post-traumatic stress disorder in people with intellectual disabilities: The development and psychometric properties of the Impact of Event Scale-Intellectual Disabilities (IES-IDs). *British Journal of Clinical Psychology, 53*(3), 315–332. doi:10.1111/bjc.12048

Harper, D. & Moss, D. (2003). A different kind of chemistry? Reformulating 'formulation'. *Clinical Psychology, 25*, 6–10.

Harper, S. K., Webb, T. L. and Rayner, K. (2013). The effectiveness of mindfulness-based interventions for supporting people with intellectual disabilities: A narrative review. *Behavior Modification, 37*(3), 431–453.

Harris, R. (2013). Material from https://www.actmindfully.com.au/free-stuff/extra-bits-ebooks-worksheets-and-handouts/ intended for use with: *Getting Unstuck in ACT: A Clinician's Guide to Overcoming Common Obstacles in Acceptance and Commitment Therapy*. New Harbinger.

Harris, R. (2019a). *ACT Made Simple: An Easy-to-Read Primer on Acceptance and Commitment Therapy*. New Harbinger.

Harris, R. (2019b). *Getting Unstuck in ACT: A Clinician's Guide to Overcoming Common Obstacles in Acceptance and Commitment Therapy*. New Harbinger.

Hatton, C. & Emerson, E. (2004). The relationship between life events and psychopathology amongst children with intellectual disabilities. *Journal of Applied Research in Intellectual Disabilities, 17*, 109–117.

Hayes, S. C. (1994). Content, Context, and the Types of Psychological Acceptance. In S. C. Hayes, N. S. Jacobson, V. M. Follette & M. J. Dougher (Eds.), *Acceptance and Change: Content and Context in Psychotherapy* (pp.13–32). Context Press.

Hayes, S. C. (2004). Acceptance and Commitment Therapy and the New Behavior Therapies: Mindfulness, Acceptance, and Relationship. In S. C. Hayes, V. M. Follette & M. M. Linehan (Eds.), *Mindfulness and Acceptance: Expanding the Cognitive-Behavioral Tradition* (pp.1–29). Guilford Press.

Hayes, S. C. (2019). *A Liberated Mind: The Essential Guide to ACT*. Random House.

Hayes, S. C. & Lillis, J. (2012). Future Developments. In S. C. Hayes & J. Lillis (Eds.), *Acceptance and Commitment Therapy* (pp.127–132). American Psychological Association.

Hayes, S. C., Strosahl, K. D. & Wilson, K. G. (1999). *Acceptance and Commitment Therapy: An Experiential Approach to Behavior Change*. Guilford Press.

Hayes, S. C., Strosahl, K. D. & Wilson, K. G. (2011). *Acceptance and Commitment Therapy: The Process and Practice of Mindful Change* (2nd edn). Guilford Press.

Hayes, S. C., Vilatte, M., Levin, M. & Hilderbrandt, M. (2011). Open, aware and active: Contextual approaches as an emerging trend in the behavioural and cognitive therapies. *Annual Review of Clinical Psychology, 7*, 141–168.

Hayes, S. C., Pistorello, J. & Levin, M. E. (2012). Acceptance and commitment therapy as a unified model of behavior change. *The Counseling Psychologist, 40*(7), 976–1002.

Heider, F. (1958). *The Psychology of Interpersonal Relations.* John Wiley & Sons.

Heslop, P., Blair, P., Fleming, P., Hoghton, M., Marriott, A. & Russ, L. (2013). *Confidential Inquiry into Premature Deaths of People with Learning Disabilities (CIPOLD).* Norah Fry Research Centre.

Hoboubi, N., Choobineh, A., Kamari Ghanavati, F., Keshavarzi, S. & Hosseini, A. A. (2017). The impact of job stress and job satisfaction on workforce productivity in an Iranian petrochemical industry. *Safety and Health at Work, 8*(1), 67–71.

Hofmann, S. G. & Hayes, S. C. (2019). The future of intervention science: Process-based therapy. *Clinical Psychological Science, 7*(1), 37–50.

Hollocks, M. J., Lerh, J. W., Magiati, I., Meiser-Stedman, R. & Brugha, T.S. (2019). Anxiety and depression in adults with autism spectrum disorder: A systematic review and meta-analysis. *Psychological Medicine, 49*(4), 559–572.

Iacoviello, B. M. & Charney, D. S. (2014). Psychosocial facets of resilience: Implications for preventing posttrauma psychopathology, treating trauma survivors, and enhancing community resilience. *European Journal of Psychotraumatology, 5.* doi:10.3402/ejpt.v5.23970

Inclusion London. (2015). *Annual Report 2014–2015.* www.inclusionlondon.org.uk/wp-content/uploads/2015/11/InclusionLondonAnnualReport2014-15_small.pdf

Jahoda, A., Hastings, R., Hatton, C., Cooper, S. A. et al. (2017). Comparison of behavioural activation with guided self-help for treatment of depression in adults with intellectual disabilities: A randomised controlled trial. *The Lancet Psychiatry, 4*(12), 909–919.

Jahoda, A., Dagnan, D., Hastings, R., Gilhooly, A. et al. (2024). Adapting psychological interventions for people with severe and profound intellectual disabilities: A behavioural activation exemplar. *Journal of Applied Research in Intellectual Disabilities, 37*(2), e13199.

Jimenez, R., Andersen, S., Song, H. & Townsend, C. (2021). Vicarious trauma in mental health care providers. *Journal of Interprofessional Education & Practice, 24*(1), 100451.

Johnstone, L. & Boyle, M. (2018). The Power Threat Meaning Framework: An alternative nondiagnostic conceptual system. *Journal of Humanistic Psychology* [Advance online publication]. doi:10.1177/0022167818793289

Johnstone, L. & Dallos, R. (Eds.) (2006). *Formulation in Psychology and Psychotherapy: Making Sense of People's Problems.* Routledge.

Jones, R. S. P. & Williams, J. (2023). *The Art of Caring for People with Intellectual Disabilities.* Pavilion.

Keijsers, G. P., Schaap, C. P. & Hoogduin, C. A. (2000). The impact of interpersonal patient and therapist behaviour on outcome in cognitive behavioural therapy. A review of empirical studies. *Behaviour Modification, 24*(2), 264–297.

Kinnaird, E., Stewart, C. & Tchanturia, K. (2019). Investigating alexithymia in autism: A systematic review and meta-analysis. *European Psychiatry, 55*, 80–89.

Konstantinou, P., Ioannou, M., Melanthiou, D., Georgiou, K. et al. (2023). The impact of acceptance and commitment therapy (ACT) on quality of life and symptom improvement among chronic health conditions: A systematic review and meta- analysis. *Journal of Contextual Behavioral Science, 29*, 240–253. doi:10.1016/j.jcbs.2023.08.004

Ledger, S., McCormack, N., Walmsley, J., Tilley, E. & Davies, I. (2022). 'Everyone has a story to tell': A review of life stories in learning disability research and practice. *British Journal of Learning Disabilities, 50*(4), 484–493.

Leoni, M., Corti, S. & Cavagnola, R. (2015). Third generation behavioural therapy for neurodevelopmental disorders: Review and trajectories. *Advances in Mental Health and Intellectual Disabilities, 9*(5), 265–274.

Leoni, M., Corti, S., Cavagnola, R., Healy, O. & Noone, S. J. (2016). How acceptance and commitment therapy changed the perspective on support provision for staff working with intellectual disability. *Advances in Mental Health and Intellectual Disabilities, 10*(1), 59–73.

Levitas, A. S. & Gilson, S. F. (2001). Predictable crises in the lives of people with mental retardation. *Mental Health Aspects of Developmental Disabilities, 4*(3), 89–100.

Linehan, M. M. (1993). *Cognitive-Behavioral Treatment of Borderline Personality Disorder.* Guilford Press.

Lodha, S. & Gupta, R. (2022). Mindfulness, attentional networks, and executive functioning: A review of interventions and long-term meditation practice. *Journal of Cognitive Enhancement, 6*(4), 531–548.

Lovett, H (1996). *Learning to Listen: Positive Approaches and People with Difficult Behaviour.* Jessica Kinglsey Publishers.

Macneil, C., Hasty, M., Conus, P. & Berk, M. (2012). Is diagnosis enough to guide interventions in mental health? Using case formulation in clinical practice. *BMC Medicine. 10*(111). doi:10.1186/1741-7015-10-111

Marshall, K. & Willoughby-Booth, S. (2007). Modifying the clinical outcomes in routine evaluation measure for use with people who have a learning disability. *British Journal of Learning Disabilities, 35*(2), 107–112.

Maslow, A. H. (1943). A theory of human motivation. *Psychological Review, 50*(4), 370.

Maslow, A. & Lewis, K. J. (1987). Maslow's hierarchy of needs. *Salenger Incorporated, 14*(17), 987–990.

McCarthy, M., Bates, C., Elson, N., Hunt, S., Milne-Skillman, K. & Forrester-Jones, R. (2022). 'Love makes me feel good inside and my heart is fixed': What adults with intellectual disabilities have to say about love and relationships. *Journal of Applied Research in Intellectual Disabilities, 35*(4), 955–965.

Mencap (n.d.). Health inequalities. www.mencap.org.uk/learning-disability-explained/research-and-statistics/health/health-inequalities

Mills, R., Nathan, R., Soper, P., Michelet, F., Stewart, A. G. & Jaydeokar, S. (2023). Intellectual disability and autism in adults influence psychological treatments for mental health comorbidities. *Advances in Mental Health and Intellectual Disabilities, 17*(2), 61–72.

Milton, D. E. (2012). On the ontological status of autism: The 'double empathy problem'. *Disability & Society, 27*, 883–887.

Morris, E. M. J. & Bilich-Eric, L. (2017). A framework to support experiential learning and psychological flexibility in supervision: SHAPE. *Australian Psychologist, 52*(2), 104–113.

Murphy, J. J. & Davis, M. W. (2005). Video exceptions: An empirical case study involving a child with developmental disabilities. *Journal of Systematic Therapies, 24*, 66–79.

National Collaborating Centre for Mental Health. (2015). *Challenging Behaviour and Learning Disabilities: Prevention and Interventions for People with Learning Disabilities Whose Behaviour Challenges.* NICE Guideline (NG11).

NHS England. (2021). *Learning Disability Mortality Review (LeDeR): Action from Learning Report 2020/21.* www.england.nhs.uk/publication/leder-action-from-learning-report-2021

NHS England. (2023). *Learning from Lives and Deaths – People with a Learning Disability and Autistic People (LeDeR): Action from Learning Report 2022/23.* https://leder.nhs.uk/images/resources/action-from-learning-report-22-23/20231019_LeDeR_action_from_learning_report_FINAL.pdf

NICE (National Institute for Health and Care Excellence). (2018). *Post-traumatic stress disorder.* NICE Guideline (NG116). https://www.nice.org.uk/guidance/NG116

NICE (National Institute for Health and Care Excellence). (2021). Overview. *Chronic pain (primary and secondary) in over 16s: Assessment of all chronic pain and management of chronic primary pain.* NICE Guideline (NG193). www.nice.org.uk/guidance/NG193

NICE (National Institute for Health and Care Excellence) (2022). *Depression in Adults: Treatment and Management.* NICE Guideline (NG 222). www.nice.org.uk/guidance/ng222/chapter/recommendations

Nixon, M., Thomas, S. D. M., Daffern, M. & Ogloff, J. R. P. (2017). Estimating the risk of crime and victimisation in people with intellectual disability: A data linkage study. *Social Psychiatry and Psychiatric Epidemiology, 52*, 617–626.

Noone, S. J. & Hastings R. P. (2009). Building psychological resilience in support staff caring for people with intellectual disabilities: Pilot evaluation of an acceptance-based intervention. *Journal of Intellectual Disabilities, 13*(1), 43–53.

Noone, S. J., Jones, R. S. & Hastings, R. P. (2006). Care staff attributions about challenging behaviors in adults with intellectual disabilities. *Research in Developmental Disabilities, 27*(2), 109–120.

Nummenmaa, L., Glerean, E., Hari, R. & Hietanen, J. K. (2014). Bodily maps of emotions. *Proceedings of the National Academy of Sciences, 111*(2), 646–651.

Nyashanu, M., Pfende, F. & Ekpenyong, M. (2020). Exploring the challenges faced by frontline workers in health and social care amid the COVID-19 pandemic: Experiences of frontline workers in the English Midlands region, UK. *Journal of Interprofessional Care, 34*(5), 655–661.

Oathamshaw, S. C. & Haddock, G. (2006). Do people with intellectual disabilities and psychosis have the cognitive skills required to undertake cognitive behavioural therapy? *Journal of Applied Research in Intellectual Disabilities, 19*(1), 35–46.

Oliver, M. (2020, November). The development and initial evaluation of the Psychological Flexibility Questionnaire. Paper presented at the UK and Republic of Ireland ACT and CBS 4th Conference.

Oliver, M. A., Selman, M., Brice, S. & Alegbo, R. (2019). Two cases of acceptance and commitment therapy leading to rapid psychological improvement in people with intellectual disabilities. *Advances in Mental Health and Intellectual Disabilities, 13*(6), 257–267.

Ost, L. G. (2014). The efficacy of acceptance and commitment therapy: An updated systematic review and meta-analysis. *Behaviour Research and Therapy, 61*, 105–121. doi:10.1016/j.brat.2014.07.018

Ostrom, E. (2012). *The Future of the Commons: Beyond Market Failure and Government Regulation.* Institute of Economic Affairs.

Ostrom, E. (2015). *Governing the Commons: The Evolution of Institutions for Collective Action* (2nd edn). Cambridge University Press.

Osugo, M. & Cooper, S. A. (2016). Interventions for adults with mild intellectual disabilities and mental ill-health: A systematic review. *Journal of Intellectual Disability Research, 60*(6), 615–622.

Padmanabhan, S. (2021). The impact of locus of control on workplace stress and job satisfaction: A pilot study on private-sector employees. *Current Research in Behavioral Sciences, 2*, 100026.

Pankey, J. & Hayes, S. C. (2003). Acceptance and commitment therapy for psychosis. *International Journal of Psychology and Psychological Therapy, 3*, 311–328.

Pankey, J. & Hayes, S. C. (2008) *Acceptance and Commitment Therapy with Dually Diagnosed Individuals.* University of Nevada, Reno.

Peterson, A. L. (2021). Do you have dead people goals? Mental Health @ Home. https://mentalhealthathome.org/2021/03/15/dead-people-goals

Pohar, R. & Argáez, C. (2017). *Acceptance and Commitment Therapy for Post-Traumatic Stress Disorder, Anxiety, and Depression: A Review of Clinical Effectiveness.* Canadian Agency for Drugs and Technologies in Health.

Reichman, N. E., Corman, H., Noonan, K. & Jiménez, M. E. (2018). Infant health and future childhood adversity. *Maternal and Child Health Journal, 22*, 318–326.

Rogers, C. R. (1957). The necessary and sufficient conditions of therapeutic personality change. *Journal of Consulting Psychology, 21*(2), 95–103.

Rong, Y., Yang, C. J., Jin, Y. & Wang, Y. (2021). Prevalence of attention-deficit/hyperactivity disorder in individuals with autism spectrum disorder: A meta-analysis. *Research in Autism Spectrum Disorders, 83*, 101759.

Roy, A., Matthews, H., Clifford, P., Fowler, V. & Martin, D. M. (2002). Health of the Nation Outcome Scales for People with Learning Disabilities (HoNOS-LD). *British Journal of Psychiatry, 180*(1), 61–66.

Royal College of Psychiatrists, British Psychological Society, & Royal College of Speech and Language Therapists (2007). *Challenging Behaviour: A Unified Approach (CR144)*. Royal College of Psychiatrists.

Rydzewska, E., Hughes-McCormack, L. A., Gillberg, C., Henderson, A. et al. (2018). Prevalence of long-term health conditions in adults with autism: Observational study of a whole country population. *BMJ Open, 8*(8), e023945.

Segal, Z., Williams, M. & Teasdale, J. (2012). *Mindfulness-Based Cognitive Therapy for Depression.* Guilford Press.

Shackleton, A. (2016). Have a Heart: Helping Services to Provide Emotionally Aware Support. In H. K. Fletcher, A. Flood & D. J. Hare (Eds.), *Attachment in Intellectual and Developmental Disability: A Clinician's Guide to Practice and Research* (pp.172–196). Wiley.

Sheehan, R., Hassiotis, A., Walters, K., Osborn, D., Strydom, A. & Horsfall, L. (2015). Mental illness, challenging behaviour, and psychotropic drug prescribing in people with intellectual disability: UK population based cohort study. *BMJ, 351*, h4326.

Simoes, G. & Silva, R. (2021). The emerging role of acceptance and commitment therapy as a way to treat trauma and stressor related disorders. *BJPsych Open, 7*(Suppl 1), S290–S290.

Singh, N. N. & Jackman, M. M. (2017). Teaching Individuals with Developmental and Intellectual Disabilities. In *Resources for Teaching Mindfulness: An International Handbook* (pp.287–305). Springer International.

Singh, N. N., Wechsler, H. A., Curtis, W. J., Sabaawi, M., Myers, R. E. & Singh, S. D. (2002). Effects of role-play and mindfulness training on enhancing the family friendliness of the admissions treatment team process. *Journal of Emotional and Behavioral Disorders, 10*(2), 90–98.

Singh, N. N., Wahler, R. G., Adkins, A. D., Myers, R. E. & Mindfulness Research Group. (2003). Soles of the feet: A mindfulness-based self-control intervention for aggression by an individual with mild mental retardation and mental illness. *Research in Developmental Disabilities, 24*(3), 158–169.

Singh, N. N., Lancioni, G. E., Winton, A. S., Wahler, R. G., Singh, J. & Sage, M. (2004). Mindful caregiving increases happiness among individuals with profound multiple disabilities. *Research in Developmental Disabilities, 25*(2), 207–218.

Singh, N. N., Lancioni, G. E., Winton, A. S., Fisher, B. C. et al. (2006). Mindful parenting decreases aggression, noncompliance, and self-injury in children with autism. *Journal of Emotional and Behavioral Disorders, 14*(3), 169–177.

Singh, N. N., Lancioni, G. E., Wahler, R. G., Winton, A. S. & Singh, J. (2008). Mindfulness approaches in cognitive behavior therapy. *Behavioural and Cognitive Psychotherapy, 36*(6), 659–666.

Singh, N. N., Lancioni, G. E., Winton, S. W., Adkins, D. & Singh, J. (2009). Mindful staff can reduce the use of physical restraints when providing care to individuals with intellectual disabilities. *Journal of Applied Research in Intellectual Disabilities, 22*(2), 194–202.

Singh, N. N., Lancioni, G. E., Winton, A. S., Singh, J., Singh, A. N. & Singh, A. D. (2011). Peer with intellectual disabilities as a mindfulness-based anger and aggression management therapist. *Research in Developmental Disabilities, 32*(6), 2690–2696.

Singleton, N., Bumpstead, R., O'Brien, M., Lee, A. & Meltzer, H. (2001). *Psychiatric Morbidity among Adults Living in Private Households, 2000.* The Stationery Office.

Skirrow, P. & Hatton, C. (2007). 'Burnout' amongst direct care workers in services for adults with intellectual disabilities: A systematic review of research findings and initial normative data. *Journal of Applied Research in Intellectual Disabilities, 20*(2), 131–144.

Spurrell, M., Potts, L. & Shaw, A. (2019). The Complex Case and Recovery Management framework: The CCaRM. Keynote presentation at the International Conference on the

Care and Treatment of Offenders with an Intellectual Disability and/or Developmental Disability, 10–11 April. Birmingham, UK.

Spurrell, M., Potts, L. & Shaw, A. (2023). Framing value based healthcare in practice: Introducing the Complex Case and Recovery Management Framework (the CCaRM). *International Journal of Integrated Care, 23*(1) 1–10.

Sturmey, P. (2004). Cognitive therapy with people with intellectual disabilities: A selective review and critique. *Clinical Psychology & Psychotherapy: An International Journal of Theory & Practice, 11*(4), 222–232.

Taheri, A., Perry, A. & Minnes, P. (2016). Examining the social participation of children and adolescents with intellectual disabilities and autism spectrum disorder in relation to peers. *Journal of Intellectual Disability Research, 60*(5), 435–443.

Taylor, J. L. (2019). Delivering the Transforming Care programme: A case of smoke and mirrors? *BJPsych Bulletin, 43*(5), 201–203.

Tirch, D., Schoendorff, B. & Silberstein, L. R. (2014). *The ACT Practitioner's Guide to the Science of Compassion: Tools for Fostering Psychological Flexibility*. New Harbinger.

Tomlinson, S. (2007). Network training workshops: Facilitators' and participants' views of systemic workshops in learning disability services. Thesis submitted to the Doctorate in Clinical Psychology, University of Wales, Cardiff.

Towey-Swift, K. D., Lauvrud, C. & Whittington, R. (2022). Acceptance and commitment therapy (ACT) for professional staff burnout: A systematic review and narrative synthesis of controlled trials. *Journal of Mental Health, 32*(2), 452–464.

Viswesvaran, C., Sanchez, J. I. & Fisher, J. (1999). The role of social support in the process of work stress: A meta-analysis. *Journal of Vocational Behavior, 54*(2), 314–334.

Webster, G. (2023). *This Is Me*. Scholastic.

Wigham, S., Hatton, C. & Taylor, J. L. (2011). The Lancaster and Northgate Trauma Scales (LANTS): The development and psychometric properties of a measure of trauma for people with mild to moderate intellectual disabilities. *Research in Developmental Disabilities, 32*(6), 2651–2659.

Williams, C. H. (2015). Improving access to psychological therapies (IAPT) and treatment outcomes: Epistemological assumptions and controversies. *Journal of Psychiatric Mental Health Nursing, 22*(5), 344–351. doi:10.1111/jpm.12181

Williams, J. & Jones, R. S. P. (2022). *Living Your Best Life: Acceptance-Based Guided Self-Help for People with Intellectual Disabilities*. Pavilion.

Willner, P. (2009). Psychotherapeutic interventions in learning disability: Focus on cognitive behavioural therapy and mental health. *Psychiatry, 8*, 416–419.

Willner, P. & Tomlinson, S. (2007). *Journal of Applied Research in Intellectual Disabilities, 20*(6), 553–562.

Willner, P., Rose, J. & Jahoda, A. (2014). Outcomes of a cluster-randomized controlled trial of a group-based cognitive behavioural anger-management intervention for people with mild to moderate intellectual disabilities. *British Journal of Psychiatry, 203*, 288–296.

Wilson, D. S. & Sober, E. (1994). Reintroducing group selection to the human behavioral sciences. *Behavioral and brain sciences, 17*(4), 585–608.

Wilson, K. G. & DuFrene, T. (2009). *Mindfulness for Two: An Acceptance and Commitment Therapy Approach to Mindfulness in Psychotherapy*. New Harbinger.

Wilson, K. G., Flynn, M. K., Bordieri, M., Nassar, S., Lucas, N. & Whiteman, K. (2012). Acceptance and Cognitive Behavior Therapy. In W. T. O'Donohue & J. E. Fisher (Eds.), *Cognitive Behavior Therapy: Core Principles for Practice* (pp.377–398). John Wiley & Sons.

Wilson, P. & Long, I. (2018). *The Big Book of Blob Trees* (2nd edn). Routledge.

Wolfensberger, W. P., Nirje, B., Olshansky, S., Perske, R. & Roos, P. (1972). *The Principle of Normalization in Human Services*. National Institute on Mental Retardation, Toronto.

Zettle, R. D. (2016). The Self in Acceptance and Commitment Therapy. In M. Kyrios, R. Moulding, G. Doron, S. S. Bhar, M. Nedeljkovic & M. Mikulincer (Eds.), *The Self in Understanding and Treating Psychological Disorders* (pp.50–58). Cambridge University Press.

Zettle, R. D. & Rains, J. C. (1989). Group cognitive and contextual therapies in treatment of depression. *Journal of Clinical Psychology, 45*(3), 436–445.

Zettle, R. D., Rains, J. C. & Hayes, S. C. (2011). Processes of change in acceptance and commitment therapy and cognitive therapy for depression: A mediation reanalysis of Zettle and Rains. *Behavior Modification, 35*(3), 265–283.

Zijlmans, L. J., Embregts, P. J., Bosman, A. M. & Willems, A. P. (2012). The relationship among attributions, emotions, and interpersonal styles of staff working with clients with intellectual disabilities and challenging behavior. *Research in Developmental Disabilities, 33*(5), 1484–1494.

Appendix 1:
Values Handouts and Worksheets

You can download the following handouts and worksheets at https://digitalhub.jkp.com/redeem (or scan the QR code) using the voucher code UAHJYLC.

- Values worksheet
- Values Scale I
- Values Scale II
- Easy-Read Values Satisfaction exercise
- Easy-Read Bullseye worksheet (Figure 5.1)

Appendix 2:
Putting it all together: a summary of the adapted Hexaflex exercises

Noticing		
Be aware **(Self as context)**	**Be here now** **(Contact with the present moment)**	**Watch your thinking** **(Defusion)**
Self-to-world relational frame. Exercises include: • Deconstruction of life story work • 'I can be' or 'times I am' statements • The observing self • Visual depiction of roles • Opposites • Blob figures • String and Post-it note exercise (the different roles adopted) • Supporters: the different roles played	Exercises include 'doing tasks': • Mindful eating • Dropping anchor (or 'hokey cokey') • Checking in during therapy • Noticing your own hands • Movement • Fun exercises • Music therapy • Leaves on a stream • Mindful colouring • Mindfulness apps • Soles of the feet meditation	Key points: Use visual aids and consider scenarios to clarify the concept of 'thoughts'. Exercises include: • Mindful versus mind full • Use of metaphors, e.g. chip shop, pushing paper away • Thoughts on balloons • Passengers on the bus • Singing/saying the word • Use special interests • Psychoeducation on thoughts/training in thoughts spotting • I'm noticing that...

cont.

• Supporters: teach soles of feet meditation, introduce mindfulness, debriefing using mindfulness, offer/encourage mindfulness during supervision e.g. attention to feelings • Encourage supporters to model noticing skills • Supporters to reflect back what noticed	• Thoughts versus facts • Supporters: notice attributions

Feeling	
Open up **(Acceptance)**	**Compassion skills**
Key points: Generate collaborative accessible understanding of concept. Exercises include: • Urge surfing • Emotions have a message • Mindfulness • Passengers on the bus • Tailoring metaphors to individual need • Dropping the struggle • Adopting different postures • 'Taking up space' exercises • Supporters: normalizing difficult reactions/debriefing/sit with the feeling/mindfulness of feelings	Key points: Support to foster a sense of compassion – to self and others. Exercises include: • Older, wiser self • Advice to best friend • Compassionate other • Receiving compassion from others • Being compassionate to others • Acts of kindness, e.g. volunteering, giving back to the community (linked to values)

cont.

Doing	
Know what matters **(Values)**	**Do what it takes** **(Committed action)**
'Where the rubber hits the road'	
Key points: Informal assessment of values, distress underpinned by values. Exercises include: • Framing the question creatively • Person-centred planning e.g. one-page profiles (individual and system level) • Photography • Values card sorting task • Human yearnings • Check: important to me versus others • Where there is pain there is a value • Adapted values sheets • Supporters: integrate values into PBS plans • Card sorting in relation to supporting role • Consider similarities and differences to each other • Values-based goals for appraisals/supervisions	Key points: Generate collaborative list of values-based actions. Construct list of day-to-day activities and link to identified values. Exercises include: • Kind actions/rate on bulls-eye diagram and regularly review • Behavioural activation • Enlisting support • Exposure • Practise, practise, practise! • Cue cards for goals • Create visual goals • Adapted goals sheets • Supporters: goals as part of performance reviews/supervision

Subject Index

Author Index

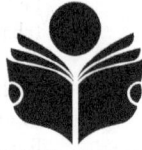

RAISING READERS
Books Build Bright Futures

Dear Reader,

We'd love your attention for one more page to tell you about the crisis in children's reading, and what we can all do.

Studies have shown that reading for fun is the **single biggest predictor of a child's future life chances** – more than family circumstance, parents' educational background or income. It improves academic results, mental health, wealth, communication skills, ambition and happiness.[1]

The number of children reading for fun is in rapid decline. Young people have a lot of competition for their time. In 2024, 1 in 10 children and young people in the UK aged 5 to 18 did not own a single book at home.[2]

Hachette works extensively with schools, libraries and literacy charities, but here are some ways we can all raise more readers:

- Reading to children for just 10 minutes a day makes a difference
- Don't give up if children aren't regular readers – there will be books for them!
- Visit bookshops and libraries to get recommendations
- Encourage them to listen to audiobooks
- Support school libraries
- Give books as gifts

There's a lot more information about how to encourage children to read on our website: **www.RaisingReaders.co.uk**

Thank you for reading.

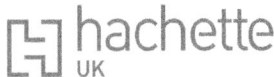

hachette
UK

1   OECD, '21st-Century Readers: Developing Literacy Skills in a Digital World', 2021, https://www.oecd.org/en/publications/21st-century-readers_a83d84cb-en.html
2   National Literacy Trust, 'Book Ownership in 2024', November 2024, https://literacytrust.org.uk/research-services/research-reports/book-ownership-in-2024